TOP 10 Geriatric Syndromes

CLINICAL MANAGEMENT STRATEGIES

Lisa Byrd, PhD, FNP-BC, GNP-BC

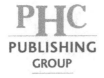

PHC
PUBLISHING
GROUP

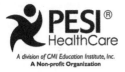

PESI®
HealthCare
A division of CMI Education Institute, Inc.
A Non-profit Organization

EAU CLAIRE, WISCONSIN
2011

Copyright © 2011

PESI HEALTHCARE
PO BOX 900
EAU CLAIRE WI 54702-0900

Printed in the United States of America

ISBN: 978-0-9845254-6-1

For information on this and other
PESI HealthCare products
please call 800-843-7763 or
visit our website at www.pesihealthcare.com

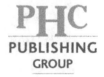

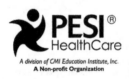

Editing: Yvonne Kuter
Cover Design: Heidi Knower

Preface

Many people are living long healthy lives, but there are many normal changes that occur due to the aging process and several common problems which present in elders. People are having longer life expectancies than in previous generations and there is predicted to be an explosion of the older population. Understanding the expected changes due to normal aging, as well as what changes are not normal, will help individuals and those who care for older individuals develop a more appropriate plan for lifestyle and healthcare. A significant number of older adults will eventually develop one or more of a group of related medical problems referred to as 'Geriatric Syndromes'. These syndromes are a cascade of problems in an elder's health and revolve around vision and hearing problems, elimination issues, dizziness, falls, and cognitive impairment including delirium as well as dementia (such as Alzheimer's disease). These syndromes can limit a person's ability to carry out basic daily activities, may threaten independence, and can diminish quality of life as well as lead to death.

Geriatrics is a specialty which focuses on care of adults over the age of 60. Geriatric syndromes are due to changes caused by aging, usually have more than one cause, and involve several different body systems. In addition, one geriatric syndrome often contributes to another. For example, the inability to completely empty one's bladder may lead to a bladder infection, which may, in turn, lead to a urinary tract infection and cause (or worsen) confusion. For these reasons, providing healthcare for older individuals with Geriatric Syndromes can be complicated due to elders' multiple conditions or diagnoses (hypertension and diabetes and arthritis) and multiple medication usage by many in this age group.

This book will present many of the expected changes caused by normal aging and the Top Ten Geriatric Syndromes elders experience. It will provide a guide to care presented in a concise, easy to utilize format of treatment strategies. It will also present a discussion of the differing presentations of illnesses in elders and encourage utilization of strategies which are age-appropriate.

The following are the top ten Geriatric Syndromes:

Fall Specialse
- Falls
- Sleep
- Pain
- Eating problems
- Confusion (dementia/depression)
- Incontinence
- Anxiety
- Living abilities (Activities of Daily Living-ADLs)
- Skin Integrity Issues
- Elimination Issues

The author brings expertise in developing geriatric-appropriate treatment strategies based on over 25 years working in nursing/healthcare, over 15 years working as a Nurse Practitioner caring for elders, and from best practices in geriatric care based on research in the field. The strategies are based on evidence-based outcomes by leading geriatric experts and an extensive search through up-to-date literature, as well as the author's professional and personal practice experiences.

Acknowledgements

Time marches on and changes occur in every individual. The baby boomers are graying and the older population is exploding in numbers. This segment of the population sometimes requires uniqueness in care to prevent problems, promote health, and diminish the consequences associated with normal aging changes. Aging is an expected occurrence in the lives of every person and this book, 'Top Ten Geriatric Syndrome' was a work meant to offer information, advice, and help those who are managing the issues I see on a daily basis in my profession as a Nurse Practitioner.

I would like to express my gratitude to the many people who saw me through this book; to all those who provided support, talked things over, read, wrote, offered comments, proofreading, and design.

Above all I want to thank my husband, Ricky and my children- Josh and Sarah. I would also like to thank my Mother, Susie who we lost in 2009. She was my inspiration as well as my mentor- her image graces the cover of this book in the shadow. She is always there watching over every day of our lives and she is the person who made me who I am as well as gave me my love for the geriatric community.

I would like to thank PESI Healthcare for enabling me to publish this book– they had the belief that I could write a book worthy of helping others. I would also like to thank Heidi Knower for the arduous process of editing and molding this into a publishable work. There is a vast amount of information available in geriatric care that could have been included but we attempted to mold this book into a concise strategic handbook.

Last and not least: I beg forgiveness of anyone who has been with me over the course of the years and whose names I have failed to mention.

Table of Contents

Aging demographics and the explosion of the geriatric population as the 'Baby Boomers' come of age. Normal changes of the different body systems caused by Aging - Vision; Hearing; Smell; Taste; Gastrointestinal System (including eating & elimination); Cardiovascular System; Respiratory System; Renal & Urinary System; Skin, Hair & Nails; Muscles, Bones, & Joints; and Mental Abilities & Cognition. Healthy Aging will be discussed briefly.

A fall can cause injury in an elder and can even lead to death from head injury or the complications of immobility related to a fractured hip or back. There will be a discussion of the common causes of falls in elders, including vision issues, mobility problems due to arthritis or balance problems, infections, medications, dizziness or syncope, and urinary incontinence. Strategies to prevent or lessen the incidence of falls, as well as diminish the complications caused by falls, will be presented in a concise, easy to read format.

Sleeping too much or too little in elders can lead to problems. This chapter will discuss causes of sleep issues, including caffeine (and products with hidden caffeine), medications (including insomnia medications which may actually lead to worsening of the problem), nocturia (getting up at night to urinate or empty one's bladder), sleep apnea, restless leg syndrome, Dream Directed Behaviors, and dementia as well as 'sundowning' behaviors. Strategies and techniques to enhance sleep and diminish sleep problems will be presented, including environmental, behavioral, and medication management.

Pain may be acute, but it is often chronic in many older adults for a variety of reasons, which can lead to a diminished quality of life. It is often caused by arthritis and can lead to immobility and falls in elders. Pain management includes paying special attention to activity, positioning, and pharmacological management. Strategies to manage pain in elders will be presented with a focus on precautions for the use of medications in elders. Geriatric dosages are encouraged, as well as appropriate monitoring of laboratory values, to prevent other complications.

Maintaining a healthy weight can be difficult for elders. A change in weight is often the first indicator of health problems in an older individual. This chapter will discuss the changes elders experience with aging that affect weight, including changes in taste, the reduced caloric requirements many experience due to being less active, and problems resulting from health conditions that affect weight, such as loss of teeth, diabetes, heart failure, and kidney disease. Constipation is a major problem for many elders and can cause a great deal of discomfort. A discussion will follow in the next chapter of the causes of elimination problems (constipation and diarrhea) and ways to manage both pharmacologically, as well as through dietary and activity interventions.

Constipation is a major problem for many elders and can cause a great deal of discomfort. This chapter will present a discussion of the causes of elimination problems (constipation as well as diarrhea) and ways to manage both pharmacologically, as well as with dietary and activity changes.

Older adults have many changes affecting their ability to hold their urine, which can lead to urinary incontinence. This problem can be embarrassing and cause depression, anxiety, and social isolation in many elders. This chapter will discuss the causes of urinary incontinence and ways to diminish the problem.

Elders can experience anxiety and irritability due to many reasons including constipation, infections, depression, cognition impairment, and a variety of other causes. Cognitive decline and dementia (including Alzheimer's disease) are not normal changes in the elderly population but do occur. This chapter will present common presentations of anxious elders, cognition issues (including the various dementias), and ways to troubleshoot and manage these problems.

A person's ability to care for him/herself will greatly impact their ability to be independent. Physical and Psychiatric problems in some elders can lead to an inability to perform the activities of daily living (ADLs) including the instrumental ADLs (doing light housework, preparing meals, taking medications, shopping for groceries or clothes, managing money, and using technology) as well as basic ADLs (personal hygiene, dressing, eating, transferring from bed to chair, voluntary control of urine and feces elimination, and moving around). This chapter will discuss factors affecting an elder's ability to maintain independence.

There are many normal aging changes to the integumentary system (the skin) which can adversely affect elders. There are many factors which can cause the skin to be more fragile, tear easily, and heal more slowly. This chapter will review many normal aging changes that can lead to problems, including skin tears, shingles, fungal infections, cellulitis, and ulcerations. A management protocol will be presented to care for common skin problems in elders.

This chapter presents a summary of geriatric care, including preventive care, such as screening recommendations and monitoring of laboratory results, polypharmacy (multiple medication usage, inappropriate medications used in elders, and drug interactions), and hints to optimize health in an older person.

Introduction

Aging does take a toll on a person's body and there are certain physiological changes that occur in all individuals as time goes by. Aging is something we cannot avoid, though many try to halt the aging process or at least slow it down, it is impossible to stop. Aging is universal; everyone ages, but we all age a bit differently. Aging is not a 'disease,' it is an accumulation of the changes that occur in an individual over time. It is a series of biological, psychological, and spiritual changes that occur in a person as time marches on.

There were 32 million individuals over the age of 65 in the United States in 2010 and this population is expected to quadruple by the year 2050 as the baby boomers gray. Our older population is healthier than in previous years and they are living longer than generations before them. And both the people who are aging and healthcare professionals must be prepared to manage the issues that arise by understanding the effects of aging, the common problems, and ways to enhance health as well as prevent problems (or at least lessen their impact). This book will present common occurrences in older adults as the aging process advances, including expected changes in vision, hearing, skin, digestion and weight, cardiovascular system, urinary system, cognition, and changes affecting sexuality. There are common problems many older individuals experience due to changes caused by normal aging – commonly referred to as geriatric syndromes.

Chapter 1

Geriatrics

Aging demographics and the explosion of the geriatric
population as the 'Baby Boomers' come of age. Normal
changes of the different body systems caused by Aging
- Vision; Hearing; Smell; Taste; Gastrointestinal System
(including eating & elimination); Cardiovascular System;
Respiratory System; Renal & Urinary System; Skin, Hair
& Nails; Muscles, Bones, & Joints; and Mental Abilities &
Cognition. Healthy Aging will be discussed briefly.

In almost every country, the population of individuals
over the age of 60 is growing faster than any other age group.
This can be attributed to several factors, including an increased
life expectancy along with declining growth of the younger
population resulting from smaller families, i.e. fewer children
being born into families (WHO, 2010). The world's elderly
population – defined as the segment of the population 60 years
of age and older – in 2010 was estimated at 650 million globally.
In 1996, in the United States – the baby boomer generation
of approximately 78 million began turning 50 at the rate of
300,000 a month. This has had a phenomenal impact on the
elder population's growth (Brock, 1996). By 2050, the number of
older individuals is forecast to reach 2 billion (WHO, 2010). And
the fastest growing segment of the older population is the 'oldest
old' – defined as those aged 85 and older.

Longer life is a sign of good health. The aging of the
United States population is an indicator of improving national
health. Preparing elders and their healthcare providers,
caregivers, and society to meet the needs of these elderly people
is essential: training for health professionals on geriatric care;
preventing and managing age-associated chronic diseases;
designing sustainable policies on long-term care; and creating
living environments to encourage optimal health and safety in
aging. 'Active aging' is the process of optimizing opportunities

for health, participation in healthy lifestyles and ensuring safety in order to enhance quality of life as individuals grow older. Active aging allows people to realize their potential for physical, social, and mental well-being throughout their lives and to participate in their communities, while providing these seniors with adequate protection, security, and care when necessary.

Our Aging Population

The growth of the geriatric population is unprecedented, without parallel in human history – and the twenty-first century will witness even more rapid aging than did the century just past (United Nations, 2010). The life expectancy of a person varies depending on the area in which a person lives but, in general, it has risen. In 1950, life expectancy was 46, in 2005 was 66, and it is expected to increase to 82 by the year 2050 (United Nations, 2010). Women currently are living longer than men by an average of 2 to 4 years.

As of the year 2000, 16.3% of the entire US population was over 60 years of age, a 12% increase since 1990 (ASCLS, 2003). In 2010, the elderly population had grown to 39 million, an increase of 17% since 2000. It is estimated there will be a rapid rise in numbers of elders between the years 2010-2030, increasing the elderly population to 69 million due to aging baby boomers. And between the years 2030-2050, the growth rate of elders is projected to increase another 14%, bringing the geriatric population to 79 million.

Aging & Characteristics of the Older Population

Aging is a process – it is universal, progressive, and unavoidable, occurring in all living individuals. Everyone will age as time marches on, but all will age a bit differently. Aging is not a disease, it is the cumulative changes that occur in an individual over time.

The elderly population is currently healthier and older than generations before them. Most elders are able to live independently and manage their everyday activities, but there are some conditions which can cause physical problems, as well as psychiatric problems, in elders including dementia and depression. In the past, many in society often considered loss of recent memory and diminished reasoning abilities as a normal expectation of aging, often referring to it as 'senility'. BUT not all older people will have these problems or develop dementia. It is NOT a normal part of the aging process; dementia is an organic disorder involving progressive loss of the capacity to think and remember caused by a pathological disease process just like other medical conditions such as hypertension and diabetes (Byrd, 2003). Normal aging does not cause a person to have problems with memory. A full medical work-up should be conducted on any older person who has problems with memory, has a personality change, or exhibits problematic behaviors – in order to obtain an accurate diagnosis, to rule out treatable problems (which, if appropriately treated, may be reversible) and develop an appropriate plan of care. The goal is to optimize an individual's quality of life and maintain, as well as encourage, as much independence as is possible.

What to Expect with Aging

Time does take a toll on the organs and body systems as individuals age and normal aging is associated with changes as well as some degree of impairment in everyone. Aging is universal but the manner in which an individual ages depends upon many factors, including heredity, medical history, degree of physical activity, and various environmental factors. With the increasing number of elders, healthcare providers must have an understanding of normal aging processes that commonly occur in order to develop a plan for age-appropriate care to promote independence, safety, and dignity for our elderly individuals.

Table 1-1. *Common Physical Findings & Potential Problems in Older Adults*	
General Appearance	**Potential Problems**
Poor personal grooming/Hygiene	Poor overall function, self-neglect or caregiver neglect, cognitive impairment, and/or depression
Slow thought processes and slowed speech	**Potential Problems** May represent aging changes but could be indicating a number of problems, including Parkinson's disease, depression, cerebrovascular disease, and/or side effects of a medication.
<u>Ulcerations</u>	**Potential Problems** Vascular disease, venous stasis, and/or can be due to pressure on a boney prominence if an individual has decreased mobility.
Poor skin turgor	**Potential Problems** Can be a result of atrophy of subcutaneous adipose tissue (fat) or could be an indication of dehydration/volume depletion.
Ears Diminished hearing or becoming 'Hard of Hearing'	**Potential Problems** Commonly due to hearing loss caused by aging changes, but could be a sign of obstruction in the ear canal such as cerumen (ear-wax) or a foreign object (such as cotton tip applicator/Q-tip).
Eyes Decreased vision	**Potential Problems** Common causes in older adults include far-sightedness (Presbyopia) which is normal expectation of aging but other changes to visual acuity can be caused by cataracts, glaucoma, macular degeneration, diabetic retinopathy, and temporal arteritis *(CONTINUED)*

Table 1-1. *Common Physical Findings & Potential Problems in Older Adults (CONTINUED)*

Mouth Missing teeth	Although an older person may retain their teeth their entire life, many older adults have missing teeth and may have dentures. Older individuals have less saliva production, which may allow food to remain on teeth and lead to dental caries, broken teeth, and missing teeth.
Decreased ability to eat	**Potential Problems** There are common changes which can decrease an elder's appetite, decrease their caloric requirements, and cause weight loss. Any decrease in weight of an older individual may indicate a serious health problem and warrants further evaluation by a healthcare professional.
Skin Skin anomalies, including aging spots and lesions	**Potential Problems** Aging spots or brown spots that develop on the skin can be due to changes in melatonin production. Skin tags are common occurrences in elders. Skin cancer is common in the aging population and any new or changing lesion should be evaluated.
Lungs Shortness of breath, fatigue, and various lung disorders including Chronic Obstructive Pulmonary Disease (COPD), Asthma, and Emphysema	**Potential Problems** Individuals with lung disease and heart failure may have crackles or wheezing and require proper management to promote their health. Any shortness of breath also may signal problems or worsening of a chronic disease which warrants evaluation and proper management by a healthcare professional.
Cardiovascular Changes Irregular heart-beat or pulse	Any irregular heart rhythm indicates cardiovascular disease, which warrants evaluation and management by a healthcare professional. Atrial fibrillation is a chronically irregular heart beat which can increase the likelihood of blood clots (potentially leading to strokes or heart attacks) and may require management with an anticoagulant medication – which may require routine monitoring of blood work.

(CONTINUED)

Systolic murmurs (extra heart sound)	**Potential Problems** If an extra heart sound or a systolic ejection murmur (S4) develops in an older adult after the age of 75, this may be a benign anomaly due to the calcification of the heart valves. If the individual is not exhibiting symptoms such as shortness of breath, swelling in the lower extremities, fatigue, or other symptoms, then evaluation by a healthcare professional is warranted to rule out more serious cardiovascular disease but no treatment may be necessary.
Carotid Bruit	An abnormal sound heard in the neck over the carotid arteries may indicate atherosclerotic disease and can make an individual at risk for a stroke. This finding warrants evaluation and management by a healthcare professional.
Diminished pulses in arms and legs	**Potential Problems** Presence or absence of a pulse in the wrist area (radial) or foot area (pedal) arteries may indicate vascular disease. If a pulse diminishes in an extremity and there is edema noted in the extremity, this may indicate a blood clot and warrants immediate evaluation and management by a healthcare professional.
Abdomen Constipation	**Potential Problems** Slowed bowel movements are common in older adults and may be problematic – an extensive discussion can be found in Chapter 5 on Nutrition, Eating, and Elimination.
Diarrhea	**Potential Problems** Some older adults may have problems with diarrhea, but this can also be caused by a fecal impaction, a watery stool going around the hardened feces mass in the bowels – a discussion can be found in Chapter 5 on Nutrition, Eating, and Elimination.

(CONTINUED)

Table 1-1. *Common Physical Findings & Potential Problems in Older Adults (CONTINUED)*

Prominent Aortic Pulsation	Any older adult who is found to have a pulsation in the abdomen or a prominent aortic pulsation could have an abdominal aortic aneurysm and this warrants evaluation by a healthcare professional.
Genitourinary	**Potential Problems**
Atrophy of the Reproductive Organs	Older adults have general changes that occur due to normal aging processes. In females, there is a lack of estrogen which causes older women to no longer be fertile, perhaps experience vaginal dryness, and potentially painful intercourse (dyspareurnia). In males, there is an enlargement of the prostate gland which can lead to urinary hesitancy and retention. Males may also experience longer time for arousal and an erection to occur, less forceful ejaculation, and sometimes a less firm erection. A male's erections may also not be maintained as long as in the earlier years.
	Potential Problems
Urinary Incontinence & Urinary Hesitancy/Retention	Many older adults have problems with urinary incontinence and hesitancy. This can indicate a disease or may be due to aging issues. A discussion on these issues is presented in Chapter 7.
Extremities Joint Pain Limited Range of Motion Problems with Ambulation	Many older adults have changes in their joints caused by degenerative joint disease, arthritis, gout, and other conditions. An in-depth discussion is included in the chapter on Falls – Chapter 2 and Pain – Chapter 4.

(CONTINUED)

Edema (or Swelling)	**Potential Problems** Some older adults have vascular disease as well as cardiovascular disease, which can lead to edema in the lower extremities. Mild edema may be a cosmetic problem, but could impair ambulation as well as lead to cellulitis and/or venous thrombosis. Increasing swelling in the feet can be an indication of worsening of heart disease. Edema in only one extremity may indicate a blood clot and is potentially life-threatening – this finding warrants immediate evaluation to determine the cause.
Neurological Abnormal Movements or Abnormal Mental status	**Potential Problems** Weakness or paralysis in an older person's arm, leg, or face, including changes in swallowing ability or changes in speech, may indicate a neurological disease or a cerebrovascular problem, including a stroke or cerebral hemorrhage. Any new or worsening symptoms warrant immediate evaluation and management by a healthcare professional.
Weakness	**Potential Problems** Weakness or paralysis in an older person's arm, leg, or face, including changes in swallowing ability or changes in speech, may indicate a neurological disease or a cerebrovascular problem, including a stroke or cerebral hemorrhage. Any new or worsening symptoms warrant immediate evaluation and management by a healthcare professional.

(Kane et al, 2009)

WHAT'S HAPPENING

The following information will elaborate on the common physiological changes in older adults and the resulting symptoms and/or diseases.

Eyes

Vision is a very important sense and, with age, a natural process occurs that reduces visual abilities. Aging commonly causes worsening of the ability to differentiate colors and may lead to problems with judging distance or depth perception (Cora, 2001). Approximately 92% of people over the age of 65 wear glasses. Visual acuity should be assessed annually with screening for common diseases in an elder's eyes such as cataracts, glaucoma, macular degeneration, and diabetic retinopathy (Cora, 2001).

Table 1-2. *The following are the changes to an older person's eyes and vision*

Vision: All elders experience some degree of decline in vision	• **Depth perception:** The cornea, the part of the eye which refracts light, becomes flatter, less smooth, and thicker making older eyes more susceptible to astigmatism. These changes can affect the ability to judge distance, including judging the speed of oncoming traffic.
Physiological changes: • Decreased speed of eye movements • Increased intraocular pressure • Decreased tear production • Increased lens size and yellowing of lens	• **Decreased ability to differentiate colors:** There is a yellowing of the lens which causes some reduction of the eye's ability to discriminate blues, greens, and violets; colors seen more clearly are yellows, oranges, reds, and black. • **Ptosis:** An older person can have loose skin on the lids of the eye. Eyelids may droop as elasticity is lost, causing the person's visual field to be diminished. • **Dry Eyes:** There can be a decrease in orbicular muscle strength causing the eyelid to stay open slightly, which can lead to corneal dryness. • **Presbyopia:** After 40 years of age, a person's eye looses the ability to adjust to close objects and this problem continues to progress throughout life, leading to a progressive farsightedness. • **Decreased Peripheral Vision:** Peripheral vision decreases, making the visual field smaller (a person can no longer see things approaching from the side as readily). • **Slower Pupil Accommodation:** Pupil size is smaller, creating a slower constriction in the presence of bright light. There is a slowing of the pupil's dilation in dark settings and a slowing in the ability to accommodate to changes in light. Older eyes need three times more light, making night vision somewhat impaired in older adults. Glare occurs more often for elders. For example, sunlight may be reflected off shiny objects or there may be a glare around headlights of oncoming cars.

(CONTINUED)

Table 1-2. *The following are the changes to an older person's eyes and vision (CONTINUED)*

	• **Glaucoma:** The anterior chamber of the eye decreases as the thickness of the lens increases. In some elders, there is an increase in the density of collagen fibers leading to inefficient resorption of intraocular fluids and increased pressure in the eye – glaucoma. • **Cataracts:** Lens opacities can develop after the age of 50 causing cloudiness in vision; this can progress to obscure vision completely. The vitreous humor, which gives the eye its shape and support, loses some of its fluid and fibrous support. • **Opacities:** Coalesced vitreous that have broken off the periphery or central part of the retina can develop and can be seen as spots or clusters of dots in the visual field. These are largely harmless, although they can be annoying. Drusen (yellow-white) spots can develop in an area of the macula and, as long as not accompanied with distortion of objects or a decrease in vision, this pigmentation is not clinically significant.

HEALTH PROMOTION: *Key things to remember about vision and elders are:*

- Annual eye examinations are necessary for aging eyes to promote safety
- More light may be necessary
- Glare may be more pronounced
- High contrast makes aging eyes function better for many tasks such as reading
- Peripheral vision may diminish
- Changing the eye's focus from one distance to another is more difficult
- Driving may be more difficult for aging eyes because shadows are more difficult to visualize

(Aging Eyes, 2006)

Ears

Hearing allows an individual to interact with others through conversation and is a key component of safety, allowing one to hear oncoming hazards. Hearing loss can have a major impact on an elderly individual's physical, social, and emotional well-being. It can cause embarrassment, interfere with a person's ability to interact with others, and increase chances of depression as well as cause some older people to withdraw from family, friends and social activities (Strong Health Audiology, 2006). Hearing impairment is a common problem in elders, with 20-30% of older people experiencing significant hearing loss (Cora, 2001). One of the most common hearing problems is presbycusis, a gradual, progressive bilateral hearing loss of higher frequencies which can lead to impairment of speech discrimination (making it difficult to hear consonants such as f, s, th, h, and sh). It is a type of sensorineural hearing loss, a disorder caused by loss or damage to the tiny hair cells in the inner ear that serve as sensory receptors. While many problems are due largely to an aging hearing system, there may be other contributing factors, including damage from a lifetime of noise exposure, disorders of the inner ear or auditory nerve, heredity, and obstructions caused by cerumen (ear wax).

HEALTH PROMOTION: *Tips to use when talking with someone who has a hearing problem:*

- Face an older person and talk clearly
- Speak at a reasonable speed; do not hide your mouth, eat, or chew gum
- Stand in good lighting and reduce background noises
- Use facial expressions or gestures to give useful clues
- Repeat yourself if necessary, using different words
- Be patient; stay positive and relaxed
- Include the hearing-impaired person when talking (talk with the person, not about the person, when you are with others. This helps keep the hearing-impaired person from feeling alone and excluded)

(Medicine.Net, 2006)

Table 1-3. *The following are changes to the ears and hearing in older adults*

<u>Hearing loss</u>: Approximately 1/3 of elders have some degree of hearing impairment. It usually occurs gradually. When there is a sudden hearing loss in an older individual, there is usually an identifiable cause such as occlusion of the ear canal (by wax or a foreign object), toxicity from a medication, trauma, brain tumor, or other disease process.	• **Cerumen:** (Ear Wax): The Auditory canal narrows and the cerumen glands atrophy in older adults, causing thicker and dryer cerumen (ear wax) which makes its removal more difficult and can lead to blockage of the canal.
Physiological changes: • Loss of auditory neurons • Loss of ability of hearing from high to low frequency • Increased cerumen accumulation • Angiosclerosis of ear	• **Presbycusis:** (Hearing Loss): The tympanic membrane becomes dull, less flexible, retracted, and slightly gray in appearance. The ossicle joints between the malleus and stapes can become calcified and lead to a reduction in vibration of these bones and thus reduced sound transmission. There is a slight degeneration of the internal parts of the ear, which leads to impaired transmission of sound waves along the nerve pathways. These changes are considered the most common reason for hearing loss in elders. Another type of hearing loss is caused by atrophy of the organ of Corti which is sensory hearing loss. Loss of cochlear neurons can cause neural hearing loss. • **Tinnitis:** Sometimes there is an impairment of the otic nerve, which can lead to a constant or recurring high-pitched tinnitus, such as clicking, buzzing, roaring, or ringing sound, in one or both ears. Causes of this problem include medications, infections, or cerumen accumulation; a blow to the head can also cause this problem. Tinnitus can be more pronounced in quiet settings.

Skin (Integumentary System)

An elderly person's skin thins with time, becoming less elastic and more fragile, which may possibly lead to an increase in bruising (MayoClinic, 2006). There is a deceased production of natural oils, causing skin to be a bit drier and more wrinkled. An older individual may perspire less, making it harder to stay cool in high temperatures. Hair may gray and thin. The nails grow at about half the pace as when younger, age spots can occur, and skin tags are common (Mayo Clinic, 2006). Sun exposure over the years is a significant factor in how fast the skin ages; smoking adds to skin damage, and both of these factors can increase an individual's chances of developing skin cancer (Mayo Clinic, 2006). Skin cancer is the most common type of cancer in the United States with evidence that 40 to 50% of individuals over the age of 60 years will have skin cancer (National Institute on Aging, 2006).

HEALTH PROMOTION: *Tips to keep skin healthy include:*
- Avoid sun exposure, especially between 10 a.m. and 3 p.m.
- Use sunscreen
- Wear protective clothing
- Avoid artificial tanning
- Check skin often for discolorations and any new moles, as well as changes in existing moles
- Use lotions to moisturize skin
- Consider necessity of daily baths-most elders need only bathe 3-4 times a week. If an older person must bathe daily-do not use a drying soap which may excessively dry the skin and lead to more skin tears

Table 1-4. *Skin Changes in Aging*	
Physiological Changes to the Integumentary System:	**Findings upon Assessment:**
• Loss of subcutaneous fat and thus loss of dermal and epidermal thickness (less padding – prominent in the areas around the eyes) • Dermal blood vessels closer to the surface of the skin • Atrophy of sweat glands • Decreased oil production of the skin • Slower skin repair and wound healing • Increased incidence of skin tags • Increased incidence of skin cancer	• Skin dryness • Itching (pruritis) • Decreased sweating and inability to regulate body heat • Increased wrinkling of skin as well as looser skin in certain areas including • Increased vision obstruction due to skin folds of eyelids • Loss of padding over boney prominences resulting in more skin pressure sites and pain • Increased time for skin tears or wounds to heal

(Kane, Ouslander, Abrass, & Resnick, 2009)

Oral Health

The ability to eat depends on an individual's oral health, mainly if an individual has teeth and the health of their oral cavity (including the gums). Elders can keep their own teeth all of their lives if they maintain good oral hygiene (Wisconsin Dental Association, 2006). Aging can cause an individual to produce less saliva (which can lead to a drier oral mucosa and slight recession of the gumline) and food may not be as readily rinsed from the teeth; these factors can lead to tooth decay, more brittle teeth, and breakage of teeth (Vissink, Spijkervet, & van Nieuw Amerongen, 1997). Tooth decay and loss are common in an elderly person, leading to eating difficulties or denture use. The presence or absence of teeth significantly affects an elder's ability to eat and oral health should be assessed routinely, including the fit of dentures. A habit of good oral hygiene can prevent tooth decay and loss.

Weight/Digestion

Maintaining a healthy weight – or losing weight – may be more difficult as one ages. Changes in weight may be an early indicator of a health problem and should be assessed promptly. Age does cause metabolism to generally slow, caloric needs are usually less and, if less active, there is an even lower caloric requirement, allowing the calories taken in to be stored as fat (Mayo Clinic, 2006). Taste buds may change as one ages, causing foods to taste differently or food preferences to change. Saliva production is decreased leading to a drier mouth and possibly difficulty swallowing (Cora, 2001). The acidity of saliva may also contribute to a dry mouth (xerostomia), difficulty swallowing (dysphagia), and difficulty digesting starches (Cora, 2001). There is a thinning of the esophageal wall and relaxation of the cardiac sphincter which can contribute to a full feeling, there is less production of gastric secretions leading to dyspepsia, and peristalsis is slower which can lead to increased flatulence and constipation (Cora, 2001).

(Kane, Ouslander, Abrass, & Resnick, 2009)
HEALTH PROMOTION: *To stay at a healthy weight, elders need to balance the number of calories with the amount they are able to burn off. Other ways to maintain health are:*
- Adequate hydration (at least 1500 cc daily unless contraindicated)
- A diet high in fiber to encourage bowel elimination
- Eat a variety of foods including vegetables, fruits, meat, dairy products, and grains that provide for vitamins and minerals
- Avoid or limit foods high in saturated fats or that are high in calories which can increase cholesterol levels
- Stay physically active and exercise routinely
- Get an adequate amount of sleep

Table 1-5. *Changes to the Gastrointestinal (GI) tract*

Physiological changes of the GI tract:	Findings upon Assessment:
• Decreased liver size • Less efficient cholesterol stabilization & resorption (increased cholesterol levels) • Fibrosis & atrophy of salivary glands (dryer mouth) • Decreased muscle tone of the bowels (more constipation) • Slowing esophageal emptying • Atrophy of the mucosal lining • Decreased gastic acid secretion	• Decrease efficiency to process medications in the liver (leading to issues with medication dosing) • Increased indigestion as well as discomfort after eating • Increased problems with esophageal spasms • Decreased calcium absorption as well as iron absorption • Increased risk of diverticular disease
Sensory changes: • Decreased number of olfactory neurons • Altered ability to taste sweet & salty foods (still intact – ability to taste bitter & sour)	**Smell:** • Decreased sense of smell • Inability to smell noxious odors • Decreased ability to taste foods due to decreased sense of smell
Teeth: • Dryer mouth allows food to remain on teeth longer with an increased risk for dental caries, brittle teeth, and missing teeth • Decreased immunity increases risks of developing gingivitis and other infections	**Eating:** • Decreased intake due to changes in ability to taste foods • Decreased intake due to dental caries, broken or missing teeth, or an oral infection

Cardiovascular System

Over time, in most people, the heart becomes less effective and must work harder to pump the same amount of blood through a person's body (Mayo Clinic, 2006). The blood vessels become less elastic, there is some degree of hardened fatty deposits in the walls of arteries (atherosclerosis), and there is a natural loss of elasticity of the arteries, making them a little stiffer (Mayo Clinic, 2006). These cumulative changes can lead to hypertension but not all individuals over the age of 65 will develop hypertension because there are other factors that influence the development of this problem, such as family

Table 1-6. *Changes to the Cardiovascular System*	
Cardiovascular System – Physiological Changes:	**Findings upon Assessment:**
• Atrophy of the muscle fibers which line the interior of the heart • Atherosclerosis of vessels • Increased systolic pressure • Decreased compliance of left ventricle	• Increased blood pressure • Increased emphasis on atrial contracture with an S4 audible (physiological anomaly, but not significant of an acute problem) • Increased arrhythmias • Increased risk of hypotension with position changes

(Kane, Ouslander, Abrass, & Resnick, 2009)

HEALTH PROMOTION: *To increase one's chances of a healthy cardiovascular status*:
• Eat a healthy diet that is low in cholesterol
• Stay physically active
• Avoid smoking (or stop smoking)
• Manage problems such as hypertension and diabetes
• Periodic evaluation of blood pressure and health status, including annual laboratory tests

Respiratory System

The respiratory system begins at the nose and ends in the small air sacs within the lungs know as alveoli. With aging, the nose elongates downward slightly, which can restrict airflow and lead to breathing problems. There is stiffening of the larynx and trachea due to calcification and the cilia lining the trachea and pharynx are less effective, resulting in more accumulation of mucous and substances from the environment. The respiratory muscles may become weaker and the chest wall becomes stiffer. These factors, in combination with a slight downward slant of the rib cages due to osteoporosis, can lead to a diminished expansion of the chest wall. Internally, the larger and more central airways increase in diameter, resulting in an increase in anatomic and physiologic dead space. Voice pitch may increase in men (higher pitch) and decrease in women (lower pitch) (Ebersole et al, 2004).

The prominent age-related change in the respiratory system is reduced efficiency. Exercise tolerance may decline leading to fatigue and shortness of breath occurring when unusual or stressful circumstances cause the demand for oxygen to surpass available supply. Older individuals may also have a lower resistance to infection due to a diminished immune system response in combination with less effective self-cleansing action of the respiratory cilia (Ebersole et al, 2004).

Table 1-7. *Changes to the Respiratory System*	
Cardiovascular System – Physiological Changes:	**Findings upon Assessment:**
• Decreased lung elasticity • Thoracic wall calcification • Decreased respiratory muscle strength • Decreased efficiency of ventilator exchanges	• Increased risk for developing lung infections including pneumonia • Increased risk of aspiration • Increased sensitivity to narcotics

(Kane, Ouslander, Abrass, & Resnick, 2009)

HEALTH PROMOTION:
- Exercise routinely
- If the lungs are congested, decrease dairy intake and increase water intake (unless contraindicated)
- Treat lung problems promptly
- If problems with sleep apnea – decrease weight and consider continuous positive airway pressure (CPAP) if prescribed by a healthcare professional
- Maintain lung health – follow the advice of a healthcare professional
- Stop smoking

Urinary Tract
Females

Most complaints by elders regarding the urinary system involve issues related to urine elimination; in females the most popular complaint is urinary incontinence. Aging does not cause urinary incontinence but several age-related changes do contribute to it. Urinary incontinence is involuntary loss of urine and is prevalent in 15-30% of elders (Reuben, Yoshikawa, & Besdine, 1996 [9]). Women experience a thinning of the vaginal walls after menopause and a weakening of the pelvic muscles, the muscles that support the bladder.

HEALTH PROMOTION: *Treatments for urinary incontinence are:*
- Kegel exercises (see chapter 7 on Urinary Incontinence Management)
- Double voiding (voiding, waiting a short time then attempting to void the bladder again to completely empty the bladder) to completely empty the bladder while leaning forward and pressing slightly on the lower abdomen
- Biofeedback
- Behavioral therapies, including bladder training
- Medications and surgeries are a last resort

Males

In males, the most popular complaint is hesitation in urination and/or nocturia (getting up several times a night to urinate). Elderly men experience an enlargement of the prostate which can impede emptying of the bladder and lead to urinary retention – causing a gentleman to have to make frequent trips to completely empty the bladder. A urinalysis and a prostate examination should be performed annually and more often in males who have urinary complaints.

Table 1-8. *Changes to the Genitourinary System*	
Physiological Changes of the Urinary System:	**Findings upon Assessment:**
• Reduced renal mass • Loss of filtration cells (glomeruli) • Decline in functioning of the kidney filtration system (both body fluids and electrolytes), filtration of byproducts (waste products) as well as medication • Decreased bladder muscle tone • Increased abdominal girth (increased waistline size) • Males have a naturally-occurring increase in prostate size – both externally as well as internally – obstructing the outflow of urine from the bladder	• Decreased fluid and electrolyte management including decreased ability to conserve sodium • Decreased clearance of byproducts such as Creatinine and BUN • Altered drug clearance • Decreased bladder size (bladder capacity) • Increased urine left in bladder after voiding (residual urine) • Increased urgency to urinate • In certain individuals – decreased ability to void efficiently (either urinary incontinence or hesitancy in urination)

Sexuality

Romance does not stop at a certain age and advanced age does not mean an individual is no longer sexually active. Often, elders are comfortable with their partners and continue to be sexually active into their old age. There are certain issues which cause changes in a senior's ability to participate in sexual activity. After menopause, women may experience a thinning of the vaginal walls, weakening of the pelvic muscles, and a decrease in vaginal secretions causing a drying of the vagina (Merck Manual, 2010). Lubricants or medications are recommended to assist in this area if this issue is problematic. Males may require a bit longer achieving arousal and penile erection, can experience premature ejaculation, or may have difficulty maintaining an erection. Many of these issues may be related to prostate enlargement, side effects of medications, or other health issues such as heart disease. Men who are sexually active and having issues may be able to lessen these problens by allowing more time for the arousal and removing the pressure to perform. There are medications available to help, if necessary and not medically prohibited. As with any age group, elders are at risk for sexually transmitted diseases and these issues must be addressed in individuals who seek sexual relations with different partners.

Table 1-9. *Changes in Sexuality and Reproduction*	
Physiological Changes of the Urinary System:	**Findings upon Assessment:**
• In females – inability to become pregnant • Males can continue to be fertile into old age, although there is decreased sperm production • Atrophy & fibrosis of the cervical and uterine walls • Decreased hormones • Breast tissue may atrophy	• Decreased fluid and electrolyte management including decreased ability to conserve sodium • Decreased clearance of byproducts such as Creatinine and BUN • Altered drug clearance • Decreased bladder size (bladder capacity) • Increased urine left in bladder after voiding (residual urine)

(Kane, Ouslander, Abrass, & Resnick, 2009)

Bones & Joints

As people age, bones shrink slightly in size and density leading to the old adage of 'getting shorter as you age' (AARP, 2004). An individual reaches maximum bone mass at 25 to 35 years of age. This decreasing density leads to weaker bones and osteoporosis, possibly causing an increased tendency to fracture from falls (Miller, Zylstra, & Standridge, 2000). Women are especially prone to osteoporosis because menopause causes women to produce less estrogen, a hormone which had previously helped protect the bones.

Arthritis is also a common ailment in elders causing pain, stiffness, and problems with mobility (Miller et al, 2000). Arthritis is an inflammation of the joints and affects nearly ½ the people over the age of 65 (Cora, 2001). It is one of the leading causes of immobility in elders.

Table 1-10. *Ways mobility and function are affected by aging*	
<u>**Motor skills**</u>: Certain chronic conditions in elders can limit mobility. Illnesses such as rheumatoid arthritis, Parkinson's disease, sleep apnea, heart disease and diabetes can decrease flexibility and reaction time, increasing the risks for falls and accidents.	• Loss of Strength: Muscles, tendons, and joints can lose some strength and flexibility with aging unless physically active. These changes can lead to a slower reaction time in response to stimulation. • Decreased Range of Motion of the Neck: Bone mass or density can diminish as bones lose calcium and other minerals, especially in women after menopause. The spine is made up of several bones which have a gel-like cushion between them. In aging, the disks gradually lose fluid and become thinner, causing the spinal column to become curved and compressed – leading to kyphosis (curvature in the upper spine giving a hunched appearance). Bone spurs can occur due to aging and overall use of the spine. The cumulative effect is decreased ability to turn one's head adequately.
Physiological changes Affecting Mobility in Elders: • Decreased muscle mass • Deterioration and drying of joint cartilage • Decreased bone mass and density	**Findings upon Assessment:** • Decreased muscle strength • Increased fractures • Loss of height • Joint stiffening and pain with movement • Balance problems

HEALTH PROMOTION:
Ways to manage the symptoms of arthritis include:
- maintain an optimal weight (obesity causes extra stress on the joints)
- maintain weight bearing exercises as long as possible (walking, jogging, or running to encourage healthy bones)
- maintain mobility and exercise (water aerobics is an option – less stress on joints)
- medication management if necessary to manage pain and increase mobility

Ways to reduce one's risk for osteoporosis include:
- getting 1,000 to 1,300 milligrams of calcium daily by eating the right foods:
  - o dairy products, canned fish with bones such as sardines, anchovies, and salmon, dark-green leafy vegetables, tofu, and tortillas if processed with corn
- not smoking/stop smoking
- taking medications that can help prevent osteoporosis

(AARP, 2004)

Mentality/Cognition

The quickness of thinking normally slows as an individual ages but thinking processes are generally not affected. Dementia is not a normal part of the aging process, it is an organic disorder involving progressive loss of the capacity to think and remember (Byrd, 2003). Dementia does affect a significant portion of the elderly population and has many causes including Alzheimer's disease, vascular disease, hypothyroidism, Parkinson's disease, and Pick's disease (Alzheimer's Association, 2006). But the most common cause of dementia in the older population is Alzheimer's disease. The incidence of Alzheimer's disease increases with age as 1 in 12 over the age of 65 and 1 in 3 over the age of 80 develop the disease (AA, 2006). Any confusion observed in an older person should be investigated. In many instances, confusion has a treatable (and reversible) cause.

Table 1-11. *Common (Reversible) Causes of Confusion in Elder*		
Anemia	B12 deficiency folate deficiency chronic kidney disease	not enough hemoglobin to carry oxygen to a person's brain
Cardiac Arrhythmias	Bradycardia	heart rate is too slow to circulate enough oxygen to a person's brain
	Tachycardia: atrial flutter atrial fibrillation	heart does not pump enough blood per heartbeat to get an appropriate amount of blood to a person's brain

(CONTINUED)

Hypotension	blood pressure is too low to get an adequate amount of blood to a person's brain
Infections	a side effect of Urinary Tract Infections (UTI) or Upper Respiratory Infections (URI) in elders can include confusion
Medications	confusion can be an adverse effect of medications such as benzodiazepines, barbiturates, pain medications, anticholinergic agents including diphenhydramine (benadryl), insomnia medications (sleeping pills – even ones elders can obtain without a prescription: over-the-counter), steroids (prednisone, solumedrol), etc
Thyroid disease	Hypothyroidism and Hyperthyroidism
Other	Brain tumor, Blood clots on the brain due to a fall, Meningitis, etc

Successful Aging

Successful aging depends not only on maintaining health but also on preventing health problems. Appropriate screening can identify and diagnose issues early when conditions are more manageable. The following outlines current screenings guidelines for older adults.

Table 1-12. *Recommended Preventive Health Screenings in Older Adults*	

Colorectal Cancer Screening	• Beginning at age 50, both men and women should follow one of these testing schedules:
	Tests that find polyps and cancer
	  ☐ Flexible sigmoidoscopy every 5 years or
	  ☐ Colonoscopy every 10 years or
	  ☐ Double-contrast barium enema every 5 years or
	  ☐ CT colonography (virtual colonoscopy) every 5 years
	Tests that primarily find cancer
	• Yearly fecal occult blood test (gFOBT) or
	• Yearly fecal immunochemical test (FIT) every year or
	• Stool DNA test (sDNA), interval uncertain

Breast Cancer Screening: Mammograms	• Screening mammograms should be done every two years beginning at age 50 for women at average risk of breast cancer *There is insufficient evidence that mammogram screening is effective for women age 75 and older, so it's not recommended for this age group unless a family history of breast cancer or an abnormality is found such as a mass in the breast, dimpling of the breast, an inverted nipple, or breast discharge*
Cervical Cancer Screening: Pap Smears	• Beginning at age 30, women who have had 3 normal Pap test results consecutively may get screened every 2 to 3 years. Women older than 30 may also get screened every 3 years with either the conventional or liquid-based Pap test, plus the human papilloma virus (HPV) test. • Women 70 years of age or older who have had 3 or more normal Pap tests consecutively and no abnormal Pap test results in the last 10 years may choose to stop having Pap tests. • Women 60 years of age or older who have had a total hysterectomy (removal of the ovaries, uterus, and cervix) may also choose to stop having Pap tests, unless the surgery was done as a treatment for cervical cancer or pre-cancer. Women who have had a hysterectomy without removal of the cervix should continue to have Pap tests

(CONTINUED)

27

Prostate Cancer Screening	• Screening tests are often part of a routine physical exam – a Digital Rectal Examination, especially in men over age 40
	• Digital Rectal Exam (DRE) annually up to age 70 – the practioner gently inserts a gloved, lubricated finger into the patient's rectum and by pressing against the rectal wall can feel the back wall of the prostate gland
	• About 70 percent of cancerous tumors develop near the outer portion of the prostate and can be detected through a DRE
	• Prostate-Specific Antigen (PSA) Test – A sample of blood is analyzed for PSA, a substance produced in the prostate gland that helps liquefy semen. A small amount of PSA always circulates in the blood. High PSA levels, or levels that rise over time, could indicate prostate inflammation, enlargement, or cancer.
	• Also recommend – screening tests because of symptoms pointing to a prostate problem
	   □ Prostatitis can elevate the PSA (false elevation)
	   □ Annual PSA up to age 50
	   □ Annual PSA recommended if an individual has a life expectancy of more than 10 additional years (Annual PSA may not be necessary if an individual is chronically ill or his life expectancy is less than 10 years due to other medical conditions)
	   □ After age 70, annual PSA is not recommended
	   □ If PSA elevated – unless >10, recheck in 2 to 6 months & watch for doubling of PSA

Annual Screenings:
  Cognition
  Dental
  Hearing
  Functional
  Nutrition
  Vision
	• Annual assessment by a healthcare professional is recommended to encourage more healthy aging in older adults
	• If symptoms develop, evaluation and management may be warranted

Annual Laboratory Screenings:
  Cholesterol
  Diabetes
  Liver Functioning
  Renal Functioning
  Thyroid Disease
	• Annual assessment by a healthcare professional is recommended to monitor for disease as well as maintain current functioning in older adults
	• Recommended at least annually: Metabolic panel (21) or a Complete Metabolic Panel (CMP), Complete Blood Count (CBC), Cholesterol Panel, Thyroid Stimulating Hormone (TSH), and if appropriate, Hemoglobin A1C (Hgb A1C) for patients with a diagnosis of Diabetes to monitor status of glucose control/management

28

(CONTINUED)

Table 1-12. Recommended Preventive Health Screenings in Older Adults (CONTINUED)

Immunization for Elders	• Annual influenza immunization • Pneumonia immunization every 5 years • Herpes Zoster (Shingles) Vaccination – One time immunization • Older adults with a history of shingles may still receive this vaccination to lessen the frequency or severity of Shingles outbreaks

*2010-U.S. Preventive Services Task Force (USPSTF); 2009 – American Cancer Society Complete list of references for this section is included in the Reference list

Chapter 1 References

AARP. The pocket guide to staying healthy at 50+. *Publication No. 04-1P001-A*. Retrieved September 10, 2006, from www.ahrq.gov

About.com. (2010). MRI and Alzheimer's disease. Retrieved February 28, 2010, from http://alzheimers.about.com/lw/Health-Medicine/Conditions-and-diseases/MRIs-and-Alzheimers-Disease.htm

Aging Eye. Retrieved October 14, 2006 from http://proxima.astro.virginia.edu/infoshts/is156.html

Alzheimer's Association. (2006) About Alzheimer's disease. Retrieved September 10, 2006, from www.alz.org

Alzheimer's disease facts and figures. (2009). Retrieved February 28, 2010, from http://www.alz.org/national/documents/summary_alzfactsfigures2009.pdf

Alzheimer's Society. (2010). Alzheimer's disease: Risk factors. Retrieved February 28, 2010, from http://www.alzheimer.ca/english/disease/causes-riskfac.htm

American Cancer Society (2010). Guidelines for early detection of cancer. Retrieved June 15, 2010, from http://www.cancer.org/docroot/ped/content/ped_2_3x_acs_cancer_detection_guidelines_36.asp

Boltz, M. & Greenburg, S. (2007). Predicting Pressure Ulcer Risks: Try This series. Retrieved June 14, 2010, from http://consultgerirn.org/uploads/File/trythis/try_this_5.pdf

Byrd, L. (2003) Terminal dementia in the elderly: awareness leads to more appropriate care. Advance for Nurse Practitioners. 11(9):65-72.

Cora, V. (2001). Elder Care. Community Health Nursing: Caring for the Public's Health. New York: Jones & Bartlett. p. 792-825. 2001

eHow. (2010). Anxiety Medications Used in the Elderly with Dementia. Retrieved March 26, 2010, from http://www.ehow.com/facts_5761746_anxiety-medications-used-elderly-dementia.html

GNRS (2007). Core Curriculum in Advanced Practice Nursing. 2nd ed. The John Hartford Foundation Institute of Geriatric Nursing. New York University.

Kane, R., Ouslander, J., Abrass, I., Resnick, B. (2009). Essentials of Clinical Geriatrics. McGraw Medical: New York.

Kennard, C. (2006). Clock Drawing Test. Retrieved February 28, 2010, from http://alzheimers.about.com/od/diagnosisissues/a/clock_test.htm

Lindsay, J., Laurin, D., Verreault, R., Hébert, R., Helliwell, B., Hill G., & McDowell, I. (2002). Risk factors for Alzheimer's disease: a prospective analysis from the Canadian Study of Health and Aging. *American Journal of Epidemiology*. 156(5):445-53.

Mayo Clinic. Aging: What to expect as you get older. Retrieved October 14, 2006, from http://www.mayoclinic.com/health/aging/HA00040

Mayo Clinic. (2010). Alzheimer's stages: How the disease progresses. Retrieved February 27, 2010, from http://www.mayoclinic.com/health/alzheimers-stages/AZ00041

Mayo Clinic. (2010). Alzheimer's disease: Diagnosing. Retrieved February 28, 2010, from http://www.mayoclinic.org/alzheimers-disease/diagnosis.html

Mayo Clinic. (2010). Alzheimer's disease: Risk factors. Retrieved February 28, 2010, from http://www.mayoclinic.com/health/alzheimers-disease/DS00161/DSECTION=risk-factors

Mayo Clinic-U.S. Preventive Services Task Force (USPSTF) 2010. Mammogram guidelines. Retrieved June 15, 2010, from http://www.mayoclinic.com/health/mammogram-guidelines/AN02052

MedicineNet. (2010). Dementia. Retrieved February 28, 2010, from http://www.medicinenet.com/dementia/article.htm

MedicineNet. Hearing loss and aging. (2006) Retrieved October 14, 2006, from http://www.medicinenet.com/script/main/art.asp?articlekey=20432

Medscape. (2010). Alzheimer's disease: Pathology and Pathophysiology. Retrieved February 27, 2010, from http://www.medscape.com/viewarticle/553256_2

Merck Manual of Geriatrics (2010). Chapter 114-Sexuality. Retrieved Online March 13, 2011, from http://www.merckmanuals.com/mm_geriatrics/sec14/ch114.htm

Miller, K., Zylstra, R., Standridge, J. The geriatric patient: A systemic approach to maintaining health. *American Family Physician*. 2000;61(4):1089-1106.

National Institute on Aging. (2010). Alzheimer's disease Fact Sheet. Retrieved May 21, 2010, from http://www.nia.nih.gov/Alzheimers/Publications/adfact.htm

National Institute on Aging. Skin and aging. Retrieved October 14, 2006, from http://www.niapublications.org/agepages/skin.asp

Peterson, A. (2004). New Treatments For Alzheimer's Symptoms: To Curb Aggression, Paranoia In Dementia Patients, Doctors Turn to Schizophrenia Drugs. *The Wall Street Journal*. Retrieved March 26, 2010, from http://www.globalaging.org/health/us/2004/alz.htm

Pollock, B. (2007). SSRI Comparable to Antipsychotic for Psychosis in Dementia. *American Journal of Geriatric Psychiatry*. Retrieved April 2, 2010, from http://www.medpagetoday.com/Geriatrics/Dementia/6632

Reuben, D., Yoshikawa, T., & Besdine, R. (2003) What Is A Geriatric Syndrome Anyway? *Journal of the American Geriatrics Society.* 51(4):574-576.

Rosack, J. (2002). SSRI Improves Behavior Symptoms In Demented Elderly Patients. *Psychiatric News.* 37(7). p 28.

Salzman, C., Schneider, L., & Alexopoulos, G. (2010). Pharmacological Treatment of Depression in Late Life. Retrieved March 28, 2010, from http://www.acnp.org/g4/GN401000141/CH.html

Senior Journal. (2006) Beers Criteria for medications to avoid in the elderly. Retrieved October 14, 2006, from http://seniorjournal.com/NEWS/Eldercare/3-12-08Beers.htm

Strong Health Audiology. Aging and Hearing Loss (Presbycusis). Retrieved from October 14, 2006, from http://www.stronghealth.com/services/Audiology/conditions/aging.cfm

Vissink, A., Spijkervet, F.K., van Nieuw Amerongen, A. Changes in secretion and composition of saliva with aging. *Ned Tijdschr Tandheelkd.* 1997;104(5):186-9.

WebMD. (2010). Alzheimer's disease and other forms of Dementia. Retrieved February 27, 2010, from http://www.webmd.com/alzheimers/guide/alzheimers-dementia

WebMD. (2010). Down's syndrome and Alzheimer's disease. Retrieved February 28, 2010, from http://www.webmd.com/alzheimers/guide/alzheimers-down-syndrome

WebMD. (2010). Making the Diagnosis of Alzheimer's disease. Retrieved February 28, 2010, from http://www.webmd.com/alzheimers/guide/making-diagnosis?page=3

Wikipedia. (2010). MMSE. Retrieved February 28, 2010, from http://en.wikipedia.org/wiki/Mini-mental_state_examination#Interpretation

Wisconsin Dental Association. Dental care for the elderly. Retrieved October 14, 2006, from http://www.wda.org/Public/elderly/myths.htm

Wright, W. (2004). Osteoarthritis management today: Minimizing pain and maximizing quality of life. *Advance for Nurse Practitioners.* 12(9):24-31.

Chapter 2

Falls

A fall can cause injury in an elder and can even lead to death from head injury or the complications of immobility related to a fractured hip or back (spine). There will be a discussion of the common causes of falls in elders, including vision issues, mobility problems due to arthritis or balance problems, infections, medications, dizziness or syncope, and urinary incontinence. Strategies to prevent or lessen the incidence of falls, as well as diminish the complications caused by falls, will be presented in a concise format.

Falls remain a prominent clinical issue in elders who reside in any setting from the community to a Nursing Home setting. Common causes of falls can be related to normal aging processes, including poor eyesight compounded by poor lighting or fall hazards such as throw rugs making an elder more likely to trip and slip; physical issues affecting balance and gait, including arthritis, strokes, and neuropathy; and cognitive issues which can causing an older person to be unable to realize their physical limitations. Medications may contribute to an older person being at an increased risk for falls due to potential side effects affecting a person's balance. Certain chronic conditions can lead to increased use of medications, for example medications to manage depression, sleep problems, diabetes, and hypertension (high blood pressure) often increase an elder's risk for polypharmacy often icrease an elder's risk for polypharmacy (use of multiple medications). (AAPF, 2010)

Falls can Lead to Injury and/or Death in Older Adults

Falls are the leading cause of injury as well as accidental deaths in an older individual (Fuller, 2000). Death from falls in older persons increases dramatically with age, with falls accounting for 70% of accidental deaths in persons over the age of 75 years. Falls can be an indicator of poor health and declining function. Falling is often associated with significant disease in older individuals. Falls account for more than 90% of fractured hips, with most of these fractures occurring in persons over 70 years. Many falls occur in the nursing home setting where as many as 60% of these residents fall each year. Risk factors for falls in older persons include increasing age, medication use, cognitive impairment, sensory deficits, and dehydration. Treatment is directed at identifying and managing the underlying cause of the fall. Goals of care are to prevent falls, minimize injury related to falls, and to return a person to their usual level of functioning (AMDA, 2007).

Ways to address Accidents-Falls in Older Adults

Assess any elder who has fallen or who has had 3 falls in the last 6 months:

Begin by assessing and identifying any and all risk factors
1. Reduce any identified factors for falling
2. Initiate strength training to improve gait (ability to ambulate or walk) and balance as well as diminish fall risk
3. Continuously assess high risk individuals

See **Table 2-1. Fall Risk Factors**

Managing Falls
Steps to Manage a Fall & Prevent Future Falls

Falls can cause injury or death, and cause an older person to be more anxious about getting around due to fear of falling again. While it is not possible to always prevent falls, it is possible to put some preventive strategies in place, as well as diminish injury when a person falls, by limiting the complications associated with falls.

Table 2-1. *Fall Risk Factors*

<u>Risk Factors:</u>
- Individuals who use a cane or walker
- Individuals who have previously fallen
- Older persons who have experienced an acute illness
- Individuals who have certain chronic conditions, especially arthritis & neuromuscular disorders
- Older persons who take certain medications, especially those who use four or more prescription drugs
- Any individual who has had a significant weight loss

<u>Physical deficits:</u>
- Individuals who are cognitively impaired, such as those with Alzheimer's disease or dementia, or who have depression
- Individuals who have reduced vision (i.e., decline in visual acuity, decline in accommodative capacity, glare intolerance, altered depth perception, presbyopia [far sightedness], decreased night vision, decline in peripheral vision)
- Individuals who have difficulty rising from a chair
- Older persons with certain foot problems which affect balance, mobility, and gait (ability to walk) such as neuropathy, bunions, foot deformities, decreased sensations to feet, edema or swelling of the feet, and problems with proprioception (an inability to determine the position of an extremity)
- Individuals who have certain neurologic changes (i.e., postural instability; slowed reaction time; diminished sensory awareness for light touch, vibration and temperature; decline of central integration of visual, vestibular & proprioceptive senses)
- Older persons who have decreased hearing (i.e., presbycusis [increase in pure tone threshold, predominantly high frequency], impaired speech discrimination, excessive cerumen accumulation)

(CONTINUED)

Common Causes of Falls in an Elderly Person
- Accidents, environmental hazards-cluttered walkway, loose rugs, & anything which blocks the pathway to frequented places, or falls from bed when rapidly changing position from a lying to an upright position
- Imbalance or gait disturbance, balance disorders or weakness, pain related to arthritis and neuropathy
- Vertigo or dizziness
- Medications or alcohol
- Acute illness
- Confusion and cognitive impairment
- Postural hypotension (blood pressure dropping upon abrupt changes in position such as sitting up quickly or standing too quickly)
- Visual disorders
- Central nervous system disorder, syncope, drop attacks
- Epilepsy or seizures (either a staring seizure or seizures involving limb movement)

Drugs That May Increase the Risk of Falling
- Sedatives, including hypnotic and anxiolytic drugs (especially long-acting benzodiazepines)
- Tricyclic antidepressants
- Major tranquilizers (phenothiazines and butyrophenones)
- Antihypertensive drugs

Review History of the Fall

Fall prevention and reducing the risk of falls in elders begins with reviewing a person's medical conditions and medication history, as well as assessing for a history of previous falls. Ask if a person has fallen previously– ask both the older person and anyone who may have witnessed a fall, such as family, friends, or caregivers. Obtain as much detail as possible about a fall – the circumstances surrounding the incident, including the time of day, any possible causes, medicine use, if a fall is related to getting up quickly, or any other pertinent information; this can help developing a fall prevention plan.

Assessment of Risks

Regardless of whether or not an individual has a history of falling, it is important to identify any older person who has any risk factors which may make the person more likely to potentially fall. Evaluate medications or combinations of medications that could make someone likely to fall. For example, the use of three or more medications simultaneously increases a person's fall risk (AMDA, 2007). In addition, many medications can cause side effects which can lead to a fall caused by weakness, dizziness, lethargy, unsteady gait, confusion, or other effects. There are numerous medical problems that may place someone at risk for falling, including diagnoses that affect balance, such as Cerebrovascular disease, strokes, Parkinson's disease, neuropathy, and arthritis. Additional risks include individuals who experience light-headedness or syncope, as well as those who have complaints of dizziness or vertigo; cardiac diseases can cause someone to fall, as can orthostatic hypotension (blood pressure decreases when a person changes position such as standing)– assess heart rate and rhythm and measure the Blood Pressure in two positions (i.e. sitting and standing OR lying and sitting).

OTHER SUGGESTED SCREENING: assess for impaired vision, such as cataracts, glaucoma, macular degeneration), sensory deficits such as paresthesia (numbness in an extremity) or peripheral neuropathies, muscle strength, poor reflexes or slowed reaction times, and motor and cerebellar function.

Also screen for functional factors that can increase an individual's fall risk. Evidence of deconditioning (decreased activity tolerance) may suggest significant underlying medical problems and/or disease.

Urinary incontinence (leakage of urine) or urinary urgency (feeling the sensation of a full bladder followed by leakage of urine) can also present a fall risk for an older person. Establish bowel and bladder continence status, since urinary frequency and urgency can cause an older person to need to get up to void or defecate, leading to a fall.

Psychological risk factors which increase an older person's risk for falling may include confusion and impaired cognition, poor judgment, poor memory, inability to realize limitations, inability to assess the safety of a situation, and impaired decision-making capacity. Likewise, environmental factors, such as poor lighting, furniture placement, and loose rugs or exposed electrical cords, can also lead to falls in older individuals .

Assess for injury of any person who has fallen

After a person has fallen: Assess the individual for injury first, then assess vital signs and evaluate for possible pain with movement (hidden injuries), especially to the head, neck, spine, and extremities. Treatment or further evaluation may be necessary if there is any evidence of significant injury, such as a fracture or bleeding. Only after significant injury is ruled out, should a person be moved.

There may be a delay in discovering the complications of a fall, including a fracture or subdural hematoma (head injury) which may require observing the person for a period of time (usually it is suggested for 48 hours after an observed or suspected fall). Be aware of all relevant findings after a fall including vital signs, pain, swelling, bruising, decreased mobility, and level of consciousness.

Analyze a Fall: *What Caused it?*

Analyze an older individual's risks for falls in more detail after the fact of the fall, including the specific nature of the fall, how frequently falls are occurring, and any possible causes. It is important to differentiate between falls that occur when an elder has rapidly changed positions and falls that occur when an elder is trying to stand or ambulate – these types of falls will generally have different causes.

The nature of a fall refers to its characteristics and related circumstances. Frequency refers to the intervals between falls or between the occurrence of situations that present a risk for causing a person to fall.

Look for patterns and trends in falls. Often, falls are isolated events. It is reasonable to do a more limited screening in an older person after only one fall, but repeated falls warrant a more thorough assessment for the cause of the person falling.

If the causes of a fall cannot be easily identified and if the fall is accompanied by other signs and symptoms including confusion, sleepiness, or lethargy – it is possible that the fall is a symptom of another problem – either an underlying acute medical condition or a change in a chronic condition.

Define problems, injuries, or complications of falls and significant potential complications. Complications can include pain, fracture, bruising, bleeding, and anxiety as well as fear (including decreased ambulation due to fear of falling again). Individuals with osteoporosis (decreased bone mass) are at greater risk for fractures, even with small falls with minimal impact.

Treat the Person
Create an individualized plan of care for each older person who falls since the causes of falling are often unique to each older individual. Prioritize approaches to managing the risk for falling to prevent falls as well as minimize injuries if the person falls again. If a systematic evaluation of an individual's risk for falls identifies various potential interventions, it is reasonable to devise a plan of care that is targeted to specific risks. For example, if a person has an unsteady walk or gait, encourage the person to use an assistive device such as a walker or cane. Consider evaluating medications and make attempts to taper or stop a medication that is suspected of causing a fall or dizziness.

Use Specific Interventions aimed at managing the cause of the fall
Use specific interventions and treatments for underlying medical conditions and disorders. It is essential to identify specific

causes and determine whether treatment of an underlying cause is more appropriate.

Because many medications can cause or contribute to falls in older persons, a review of an individual's medication regimen may be necessary; adjust doses or consider stopping medications that may be associated with an increased risk of falling. It is better if this is done gradually, one medication at a time, starting with medications that are the least essential. Or consider switching to a different medication that can treat a condition or one which has fewer side effects. Implement generic approaches, such as strengthening exercises and balance training. Consider assessing the environment to decrease fall hazards.

Evaluate the Environment to reduce the risks of falling

If area rugs are in use, consider adding double-sided tape to the bottom of the rug to prevent slippage or use rugs that are secured to the floor. Assess rooms for clutter and electrical cords that cross frequently-traveled walking areas. Make sure pathways to frequent areas such as the kitchen or bathroom are free of clutter. Remember that fall mats, which cushion a individual's fall, are often used next to the bed and do not prevent falls, but may reduce the impact and thereby prevent more serious injury by providing a cushion. Bed and chair alarms are not cause-specific interventions, and may only prevent falls if a caregiver is in close proximity and can respond to the alarm.(AMDA, 2007)

Prevention is the best advice for an older individual – preventing a problem is the key to optimal health.

Table 2-2. *Interventions to Reduce the Risk of Falls in an Elderly Individual*

Risk factors	Interventions
Postural hypotension: a drop in systolic blood pressure of more than 20 mm Hg or to less than 90 mm Hg when a person is standing	• Behavioral modifications may help, such as having a person rise slowly, having a person perform exercises when changing positions (such as ankle pumps or hand clenching) and elevation of the head of the bed when preparing to get out of bed • Decrease in the dosage of a medication that may contribute to a person's blood pressure falling (hypotension); if necessary, discontinuation of the drug or substitution of another medication • Pressure stockings may assist in increasing blood return to the person's heart • In some individuals, a medication may be used – fludrocortisone (Florinef), in a dosage of 0.1 mg two or three times daily, to increase blood pressure • In some individuals, a medication may be used – midodrine (ProAmatine), in a dosage of 2.5 to 5 mg three times daily, to increase vascular tone and blood pressure
Use of a pain medication, benzodiazepine or other sedative-hypnotic drug	• Reduce use of any anxiety agents or sedative-hypnotic drugs • Use an alternative non-pharmacologic treatment of sleep problems: encourage good sleep hygiene
Use of four or more prescription medications	• Use of mild pain medications or those which do not affect an individual's gait • Tapering and discontinuation of medications causing falls
Environmental hazards for falling or tripping	• Safety assessment with appropriate changes, such as removal of hazards, selection of safer furniture (correct height, more stability) and use of grab bars in bathrooms or handrails on stairs
Any impairment in gait (ability to walk)	• Gait training • Use of an appropriate assistive device • Balance or strengthening exercises, if indicated

(CONTINUED)

Any impairment in balance or transfer skills	• Balance exercises and training in transfer skills, if indicated • Environmental alterations, use grab bars or raised toilet seats
Impairment in leg or arm muscle strength or range of motion (hip, ankle, knee, shoulder, hand or elbow)	• Consider Physical Therapy evaluation and management for fall prevention and balance testing – encourage exercises with resistive bands and putty resistance training two or three times a week, with resistance increased when the patient is able to complete 10 repetitions through the full range of motion

Improving Balance & Strength to Prevent Falls

An older person can improve their health and prevent falls as well as increase independence through improving muscle strength and improving balance. There are many ways to work an elder's muscles. Two of the most common are isometric exercise and progressive resistance exercise. *Isometric exercise* involves tensing the muscles without movement, as in pressing the leg down while someone blocks the movement. Remember though, that with isometric exercise, there is no movement – which means a person is not working on joint range of motion and flexibility; only on strength. Because there is no movement, isometric exercise can also increase a person's blood pressure (ElderGym, 2011).

Progressive resistance training is another method of strengthening the muscles. This is accomplished by lifting free weights, elastic exercise bands, or adjustable commercial cable machines. This type of exercise can be conditioned with isometric exercises. Caution should be used, since lifting heavy objects may cause injury and increase blood pressure in older adults. All older individuals should seek out professional advice before attempting a heavy weight elderly strength training program (ElderGym, 2011).

Strength Training in Elders

It is important to find just the right intensity when exercising for strength. Elders should aim for a balance between increasing activity levels and preventing injury. Generally, an older person can increase the weights they are lifting after about two weeks of beginning elderly strength exercises.

- Begin slowly
  - o Complete 2 sets of 10 repetitions in good form before increasing weight amounts (start with 1 to 2 pound weights)
- Completing each repetition in good form means
  - o Lift an object overhead to a count of 3, pause, then lower the object over a second count of 3. Wait 1 to 2 minutes between each set
- Remember not to progress if injured, have been sick, or muscles are too sore
- It is OK to begin with very light resistance or no resistance at all; progress gradually to avoid injury and minimize soreness
- Try exercising at least 2 to 3 times per week with a minimum of 48 hours between training sessions
- It is possible to strength train daily by alternating major muscle groups; for example, a person may work their legs on Monday and arms on Tuesday, etc.
- It is a good idea to obtain professional advice, though, before choosing to strengthen daily

Remember, elderly and seniors strength training can be fun, but will only show benefits if it is done regularly with the correct intensity (ElderGym, 2011).

Balance

Balance is regulated by three systems in a person's body:

- ***Visual cues*** come from a person's eyes and assist in sorting out information about the environment. An individual's eyes help see and prepare for potential dangers and obstacles, which can prevent falls.
- ***Internal spacial orientation*** tells a person where their arms and legs are positioned in space. For example, if someone closes their eyes and then lifts their arm and waves it about, they should know where the arm is because of this inner sense of feedback.
- ***The inner ear*** also contains a fluid-filled semicircular canal which gives important information on the position of a person's head and its movement in space in relation to gravity. This is why some individuals get motion sickness when there is a lot of head movement and ground movement.

When all these systems are working together automatically with the muscles, they help prevent falls and improve an elderly person's balance, so older persons can stay active and independent.

Balance Improvement & Exercise Safety Guidelines

If a senior has poor balance or is frail, there is a high potential for falls and injury – make sure they are closely supervised at all times. Ways to regain balance include:

- Progress to the next exercise when the preceding one can be done safely or if there is enough assistance to prevent falls.
- Be aware of posture. Try to maintain weight over the ankles.
- Avoid fast movements, including quick turns or changes in position.
- Use a chair as a place to perform not only seated exercise, but also to hold on to while standing. Hold on with a finger, one hand or two hands.
- Always get up slowly when rising from a chair.
- Don't close eyes when exercising or standing at a chair.
- If taking medications, ask if there are any side effects which may cause light-headedness or decreased balance.

(ElderGym, 2011)

Balance Improvement:

1. Use a chair for balancing in getting up and down
2. Consider using a cane or walker for balance
3. Use well-fitting shoes which have smooth bottoms, to prevent catching on carpets, etc.
4. Walk near a counter to hold onto for balance – the counter should be 8 to 10 feet long
    a. Walk next to counter several times a day to build up strength and balance
5. When able to tolerate additional exercises, place tape on floor to step over or add a small object to step over to further build strength and balance
6. Consider adding 1- to 2-lb weights to ankles to increase strength and balance.

(ElderGym, 2011)

Chapter 2 References

AAFP (2010). What causes falls in the elderly? Retrieved December 16, 2010, from http://www.aafp.org/afp/20000401/2173ph.html

AMDA (2007). Falls and Fall Risk Guidelines.

ElderGym (2011). Elder Strength Training; Elder Balance Training. Retrieved April 1, 2011, from http://www.eldergym.com/elderly-strength.html and http://www.eldergym.com/elderly-balance.html

Fuller, G. (2000). Falls in the Elderly. *American Family Physician*. 61:2159-68, 2173-4.

MDS 2.0. Public Quality Indicators and Resident Reports. (2010). Retrieved February 14, 2010, from http://www.cms.hhs.gov/MDSPubQIandResRep/

Sleep

Sleeping too much or too little can lead to problems for elders. This chapter will present a discussion on sleep issues as well as common causes of sleep problems in older individuals, including the use of caffeine (and products with hidden caffeine), medications (including insomnia medications, which actually can cause worsening of the problem), nocturia (getting up at night to empty one's bladder), sleep apnea, restless leg syndrome, Dream Directed Behaviors, and dementia, as well as 'sundowning' behaviors. Strategies and techniques to battle these problems and enhance sleep will be presented, including environmental, behavioral, and pharmacological management.

Sleep is the time when the body renews itself, recovers from the day-time activities, and rejuvenates. It is a time of rebalancing, detoxification, and the re-booting of the immune system. Sleep deprivation or insomnia can cause long term problems, including worsening of diabetes, heart disease, and cancers.

Sleep problems can have a significant impact on daily functioning and lead to problems affecting an older person's overall health. The most common complaints regarding sleeping issues are decreased night-time sleeping and increased daytime napping (Zec & Burkett, 2008). Sleep disorders commonly occur in the older population and are often under-diagnosed and undertreated. This issue can be a significant source of concern for caregivers of older individuals who are suffering from dementia.

There are several diverse factors which may contribute to sleep disturbances in elders. Some problems may be attributed to changes caused by normal aging or by various issues such as alterations in lifestyle, retirement, chronic health problems, changes in home life caused by the death of a relative (spouse or other family member), and changes in circadian rhythm. Changes in sleep patterns may be part of the normal aging process; however, many of these disturbances may be related to pathological processes that are not considered a normal part of aging, such as sundowning behaviors associated with dementia (Brannon et al, 2009).

SLEEPING TOO MUCH (HYPERSOMNIA)

Sleeping too much, as well as not sleeping enough, may lead to problems in elders. Excessive daytime sleepiness over a long period of time is known as hypersomnia. The symptoms are present all of the time, nearly all of the time, or most of the time. Recurring hypersomnia involves periods of excessive daytime sleepiness that can last from a short time frame (one day) to an extended time frame (several days) and may recur over the course of several years.

There are many different causes for daytime sleepiness, including the use of common substances such as caffeine – which keeps an individual awake at night, leading to daytime drowsiness due to an individual not obtaining an adequate amount of deep sleep (REM sleep) during night-time hours. Other substances affecting sleep include alcohol and certain medications. Some common factors that can lead to excessive daytime sleepiness include any behavior which disrupts the body's natural sleep rhythms, such as frequent night-time voiding (nocturia) or night-time behaviors associated with cognitive impairment (many of the dementias cause 'sundowning' – which is increased confusion and occurrence of agitation in the night-time hours). In elders, certain medical conditions, such as heart failure, chronic obstructive pulmonary disease, emphysema, etc., or use of certain medications used to manage edema and heart disease can cause frequent urination and interfere with sleep.

INSOMNIA (Not Sleeping Enough)

Insomnia affects a person's quality of life, causing excessive daytime sedation and fatigue, and can worsen other chronic medical conditions, decrease an individual's functional abilities, impact psychological status (causing depression and/or anxiety), worsen cognitive problems (confusion), and can affect a person's overall health. Sleep disorders can even hasten death especially if lack of sleep goes on for an extended period of time. Treating sleep problems in individuals with a diagnosis of dementia usually improves the overall health of the person, but care must be taken when using medications to affect sleep because they can cause problems in older individuals such as falls, orthostatic hypotension (fall in blood pressure when sitting upright abruptly or with standing), and worsening of confusion, as well as other medical problems. Treatments for sleep disorders include behavioral modifications, relaxation techniques, sleep hygiene, sleep restriction (if the person is sleeping too much during the day and has excessive energy at night-time, keep them awake during daytime) or sleep deprivation (excessively tired and unable to sleep – consider brief daytime naps), light therapy for melatonin conversion to enhance sleep , cognitive behavioral therapies, valerian (herbal supplement), Tai Chi, yoga, meditation, acupuncture, acupressure, and possibly medications, both over-the-counter as well as prescription medications (Brannon et. al., 2009). To better understand how sleep affects health, the following discussion provides a brief review of the stages of sleep, how sleep impacts daily functioning, and how lack of sleep affects the chemical balance within a person's body.

Sleep Patterns:

I. Normal sleep is organized into two distinct stages that cycle throughout the night.
   o Non-Rapid Eye Movement (Non-REM) sleep [*subdivided into 4 stages*]
     • Stages 1 and 2 – light sleep
     • Stages 3 and 4 – deep sleep or slow-wave sleep (SWS)
   o With aging, an increase in the duration of stage 1 sleep and an increase in the number of shifts into stage 1 sleep occurs

o Stages 3 and 4 decrease markedly with age and, after 90 years, stages 3 and 4 may disappear completely
II. Rapid Eye Movement (REM) sleep
   o Rapid eye movement (REM) sleep is the stage of sleep during which muscle tone decreases markedly; this stage is associated with bursts of dreaming
   o Relative amounts of REM sleep are maintained until extreme old age, when most older adults show some decline in obtaining REM sleep

Table 3-1. *Sleep Changes with Aging*		
Time in bed	Increased time to go to sleep	Older individuals spend more time lying in bed at night without attempting to sleep or unsuccessfully trying to sleep
Total sleep period	The time from sleep onset to the final awakening from the main sleep period of the day	Total sleep period increases with age because of the increase in the number of night-time awakenings
Total sleep time	The total sleep period minus the time spent awake during the sleep period	Is either reduced or unchanged in the older population compared with younger individuals
Sleep latency	The time from the decision to sleep to the onset of sleep	In women, sleep latency has been related to age increase in adults and hypnotic drug use, which decreases sleep latency
Wake after sleep onset	The time spent awake from sleep onset to final awakening	An increase occurs in the time spent awake after sleep onset in older individuals. There are a number of reasons older individuals awaken through the night – need to void (bladder distention, urinary urgency), pain caused by arthritis, restless leg syndrome, and sleep apnea or dyspnea
Sleep efficiency	Is decreased due to nocturnal awakenings	

(Brannon et al, 2009)

Older individuals spend more time in bed to get the same amount of sleep they obtained when they were younger; however, the total sleep time is slightly decreased, with an increase in nocturnal awakenings and daytime napping. Often, older individuals tend to have earlier bedtimes and have an increased time to fall asleep, but excessive daytime somnolence is not part of normal aging. Older subjects have been observed to be more easily aroused from sleep by auditory stimuli (sounds), suggesting increased sensitivity to environmental stimulation (Brannon, 2009).

Effects of Aging on Sleep
- More alert in early morning
- Drowsier in early evening
- Less REM sleep
- Less eye movement density while asleep
- The cumulative effect of sleep deprivation leads to higher evening cortisol levels resulting in:
  - Increased sleep fragmentation (more restless sleep)
  - Increased insulin resistance which can lead to more fatigue
  - Encourages/Hastens hippocampal atrophy – which impairs learning & memory

Cortisol & Insomnia
Cortisol is a natural hormone which can be affected by sleep (or lack of sleep). It is also considered a steroid that is vital in the 'fight or flight' response to stress; it is necessary in appropriate levels for normal daily living. It is needed for many dynamic processes in a person's body, from blood pressure regulation and kidney function, to glucose levels and fat building, tissue healing and muscle building, protein synthesis and proper immune functioning. Individuals with high cortisol levels often display excess weight in the middle region (an 'apple shape' body). Other effects include memory impairment, fatigue; over the longer term, these high levels can cause decreased immunity, make one's bones brittle and lead to heart disease as well as other dangerous conditions.

Normally, Cortisol is present in the body at higher levels in the morning and lower levels at night. Although stress isn't the only reason that cortisol is secreted into the bloodstream, it has been termed "the stress hormone" because it's also secreted in higher levels during the body's 'fight or flight' response to stimulation of illness, emotions, pain, as well as a variety of other stressors (Scott, 2008). Small increases of cortisol have the following effects:

- Supply a quick burst of energy for survival reasons (fight-or-flight response)
- Heightened memory functioning
- A burst of increased immunity
- Lower sensitivity to pain
- Helps maintain homeostasis in the body
- It is important for the body's relaxation response, so a person's functions can return to normal following a stressful event.

Cortisol makes a person's thyroid work more efficiently. The proper amount of cortisol – not too high and not too low – is very important for normal thyroid function, which is why a lot of people who have an imbalance in cortisol levels may have thyroid symptoms (such as fatigue) but normal thyroid hormone levels (Zava, 2011). Too much cortisol causes an elder to develop a condition of thyroid resistance, meaning that thyroid hormone levels can be normal but a person's body fails to respond as efficiently to the thyroid signal. This can lead to a slower metabolism as well as an alteration in production of certain hormones such as insulin, progesterone, estrogens, testosterone, and even cortisol itself (Zava, 2011). Insulin resistance is one example – it takes more insulin to drive glucose into the cells when cortisol is high. High cortisol and high insulin, resulting from insulin resistance, will cause a person to gain weight around the waist because the body will store fat in this region rather than burning it. Higher and more prolonged levels of cortisol in the bloodstream (like those associated with chronic stress or insomnia) have been shown to have negative effects, such as:

- Impaired cognitive performance
- Suppressed thyroid function
- Blood sugar imbalances, such as hyperglycemia and worsening of diabetes control
- Decreased bone density
- Decrease in muscle tissue
- Higher blood pressure
- Lowered immunity and inflammatory responses in the body
   o slower wound healing
- Increased abdominal fat, which is associated with a greater number of health problems than fat deposited in other areas of the body
   o Some of the health problems associated with increased stomach fat are heart attacks, strokes, and the development of metabolic syndrome

(Scott, 2008)

Cortisol is released from the adrenal glands in a pattern throughout the day. It's high in the morning (which energizes a person) and lowest levels at two a.m. (when melatonin is high and a person is sleeping). Melatonin and cortisol are inversely related, so when cortisol is down and melatonin is up, a person's body is re-energizing and regenerating. When the cortisol level stays high, a person does not produce enough growth hormone or thyroid-stimulating hormone, which will impair tissue building and healing (Zava, 2011).

High cortisol levels lead to sleep fragmentation (more problems getting to sleep and staying asleep) and sleep deprivation. Studies have shown that sleep deprivation is associated with an increase in appetite, due to the possible need for the increased caloric demands of extended wakeful periods (Cauter, Knutson, Leproult, & Spiegal, 2005). High cortisol levels can lead to insomnia – becoming a problem which feeds upon itself; i.e., insomnia causes higher cortisol levels and higher cortisol levels cause sleep fragmentation and insomnia. When a person sleeps, cortisol levels are lowered, allowing normal growth and repair of cells to take place. Without the lowering cortisol levels, a person may experience more health problems, have more weight gain, slower wound healing, more fatigue, and problems with learning and memory (Health Guide, 2010).

Other Health Problems & Insomnia *(less than 5 hours of sleep per night)*

- Individuals are more likely to suffer hypertension than people who sleep well, according to a major study that highlights the concerns over links between sleep problems and serious illness (Medical News Today, 2008)
- Diabetics are more likely to have poorly controlled glucose levels (Black, 2010)
- Even though physically equal in fitness, insomnia on a chronic basis made individuals physically weaker, have a significantly reduced exercise capacity, and a perceived greater effort during exercise (Fulcher & White, 2000)

Sleep is necessary for health and function. The body requires sleep in order to restore glycogen stores and have normal hormonal secretion. There are many factors which can cause an elder to have problems sleeping.

Factors Affecting Sleep

- Chronic conditions
  - Hypertension (47%)
  - Arthritis (46%)
  - Enlarged prostate (22% of men)
  - Heart disease (18%)
  - Depression (16%)
  - Diabetes Mellitus (15%)
- Sleep Disordered Breathing
  - Snoring
  - Apnea
- Menopausal Women
  - Menopause causes a decline in endocrine physiology and greater reduction in slow-wave activity in non-REM sleep
- Restless Leg Syndrome
  - often familial
  - inherited disorder
  - may be secondary to iron deficiency or uremia, and can be exacerbated by antidepressants, caffeine, nicotine, alcohol & inactivity
- Medication use
- Nocturia: 65% of older adults experience the need to void during night-time sleep
- Neuropsychological impairment

Other causes of insomnia
- Nocturia (waking up throughout the night to urinate)
- Going to bed too early
- Daytime napping
- Overtiredness, causing tenseness and inability to fall asleep
- Too much energy – insufficient exercise, so that the person does not feel tired
- Too much caffeine or alcohol
- Feeling hungry
- Agitation following an upsetting situation
- Disturbing dreams

Table 3-2. *Medications which can cause insomnia*
Antihypertensives
Alpha blockers
Beta blockers
Methyldopa
Reserpine
Central Nervous System Stimulants
Amphetamines
Methylphenidate
Pemoline
Decongestants
Phenylephrine
Pseudoephedrine
Hormones
Corticosteroids
Thyroid medications
Psychotropics
Atypical antidepressants
Nonselective monoamine oxidase inhibitors
Selective serotonin reuptake inhibitors (SSRIs)
Respiratory Medications
Albuterol
Theophylline
Other
Alcohol
Caffeine
Nicotine

(Chen, 2006)

Sleep Apnea

Obstructive Sleep Apnea is brief cessation of breathing due to obstruction of a person's airway, which interrupts the sleep cycle. Obstructive Sleep Apnea occurs when the support structures, including muscles and the soft tissues of the throat (the tongue and soft palate), temporarily relax, which causes the airway to narrow or close and and a person temporarily stops breathing. It is a potentially serious sleep disorder. The most noticeable sign of obstructive sleep apnea is snoring, although not everyone who has sleep apnea will snore which is the body's way of restarting a person's breathing pattern.

Anyone can develop obstructive sleep apnea, but it commonly occurs in individuals who are overweight and occurs more in men than in women. Treatment may involve using a device to keep the airway open, such as nasal strips or a positive airway machine (Continuous Positive Airway Pressure or CPAP). Another alternative is a surgical procedure to remove tissue from the nose, mouth or throat.

SYMPTOMS OF OBSTRUCTIVE SLEEP APNEA
- Excessive daytime sleepiness (hypersomnia)
- Snoring
- Observed episodes of breathing cessation during sleep
- Abrupt awakenings along with shortness of breath
- A dry mouth or sore throat in the morning
- Morning headache
- Frequent urination at night
- Difficulty staying asleep

Managing Sleep Apnea
- Lose weight
- Avoid alcohol and medications such as tranquilizers and sleeping pills, which can relax the muscles in the back of the throat, causing further breathing problems
- Sleep on one's side or abdomen, rather than on the back
- Keep the nasal passages open at night
    o If congested, use a saline nasal spray to help keep nasal passages open
    o If congestion severe enough, Medicated nasal spray may be used but should only be used on a short term basis o Consider strips to keep nasal passages open
    o Do not sleep on more than one pillow

Effect of Cognitive Impairment upon Sleep in Older Individuals

Insomnia and other sleep problems are very bothersome in individuals suffering from dementia. Some of these individuals may become more confused and agitated at night and be awake all night long wandering or performing various activities. Approximately 25% of adults with dementia experience sleep disturbances during their dementia progression (Rose & Lorenz, 2010).

Sundowning involves the occurrence or increase of one or more abnormal behaviors in the late afternoon and evening hours, which may continue into the night. It is estimated that 45% of persons diagnosed with Alzheimer's disease or other types of dementia will experience night-time behaviors (Rose & Lorenz, 2010; Wikipedia, 2010). A person who is experiencing sundowning may exhibit increased confusion, delusions, paranoia, hallucinations, and/or mood swings; they may become abnormally demanding, suspicious, upset or more disoriented. Wandering often occurs in individual who are sundowning and is the second most common type of disruptive behavior in institutionalized persons with dementia. The danger involved in night-time wandering is that person may fall, injure him/herself, or wander away and become lost.

Dream Directed Behaviors

Normally when a person is sleeping and dreaming, the muscles are essentially flaccid and relaxed (*muscle atonia*), preventing a person from acting out their dreams. But in a disorder called Dream Directed Behaviors (DDB), there is an abnormality occurring in the phase of REM sleep that leads to movement during dreams. A person is able to carry out the activities in their dreams and can become violent and/or potentially cause injury to themselves or others. The behaviors occur because a sleeping person is enacting their dream and lacks muscle atonia. The behaviors are not directed at anyone or anything in particular, though it may be that the person is enacting movements such as punching and kicking, as well as leaps and even jumps, in their bed during sleep (Sleep Disorders, 2010). It commonly occurs after the age of 60 and occurs more commonly in men than in women.

Some ways to protect a person who suffers from DDB disorder from injury include removing dangerous objects upon which the person could hit their head (such as a bedside table) from their bedrooms, clearing furniture and other objects and making sure the person cannot wander away. Consider having the person sleep with the mattress on the floor or with cushions around their bed. For individuals who have frequent problems falling out of bed (or to prevent the person from jumping out of bed) use a side-rail on a hospital bed or a toddler rail on the side of the bed. Use caution with use of loose rugs (which can create a fall hazard), and consider use of double-sided tape under rugs to prevent a person from slipping and falling if the individual rises from the bed during a dream. If a person wears socks to bed, make sure the socks have grippers on the bottom to prevent slippage and falls.

Sometimes, DDB disorder requires medications, but caution should be used because many medications for insomnia can worsen this problem and can also cause falls in older individuals. Clonazepam has been found to be very effective in treating this disorder and, in fact, success rates have been reported as being extremely high (Sleep Disorders, 2010). Non-drug treatments aim to improve sleep routine and the sleeping environment, as well as reduce daytime napping.

Improving Sleep Patterns & Enhancing Sleep
Sleep hygiene:
- ☐ go to bed when sleepy
- ☐ avoid activity in bed, such as reading, watching television, or eating
- ☐ develop a bedtime ritual
- ☐ avoid daytime naps
- ☐ if unable to go to sleep – get out of bed until sleepy
- Maintain a regular routine, including times for meals and for going to bed, as well as getting up
- A slightly cooler room is more conducive to sleep than a warmer room
- Sunlight exposure for 1-2 hours a day to enhance melatonin synthesis

Sleep

- Encourage regular exercise, but not within three hours before bedtime
- Avoid alcohol, caffeine and nicotine
- Treat pain
- If a person is taking a cholinesterase inhibitor (tacrine, donepezil, rivastigmine or galantamine), monitor if the medication seems to make the person sleepy – if so, give at bedtime; if the medication stimulates the person, then administer it in the morning
- Provide nightlights and keep the room free of clutter to prevent injury [if the person gets out of bed at night]
- If a person awakens, discourage staying in bed while awake; i.e., encourage them to use the bed only for sleep – do not eat in bed, watch television in bed, or read in bed

Food and drink

- Cut down on or eliminate the use of caffeine (coffee, cola, tea, chocolate) during the day and cut out its use altogether after 3 p.m.
- Cut down on or eliminate the use of alcohol
- If the person is hungry at night, try a light snack just before bed or when they wake up
- Herbal teas and warm milk may be helpful
- Avoid high sugar and high carbohydrate foods 3 hours before bedtime

Daily routines

- Avoid any activities that may be upsetting to the person in the late afternoon
- If the person refuses to go to bed, try offering alternatives such as sleeping on the sofa
- If the person wanders at night, consider allowing this, but make sure the environment is safe
- Try a back rub before bed or during the wakeful period
- Try a repetitive sound, such as softly playing music, beside the bed or use background noise devices such as a ticking clock
- Gently remind the person that it is night-time and time for sleep

Enhancing Sleep

- Arrange a medical check-up to identify and treat physical symptoms
- Treat pain with an analgesic at bedtime
- Screen for depression; treat, if necessary
- Consider the possible side effects of medications that may be causing sleep problems
- Consider environmental factors

Other considerations in individuals with cognitive impairment or dementia

Sleep problems, as well as late evening agitation, are often a stage in dementia that is bothersome, difficult to manage, and potentially dangerous if an elder falls or wanders outside at night.

Many individuals with dementia sleep more during the later or advanced stages of their illness. Sleep problems are among the most difficult symptoms of dementia for caregivers, who must be able to get adequate sleep themselves (Better Health Channel, 2010).

Environmental Causes of Sleep Problems in Individuals with Dementia

Sleeping problems may be caused by environmental causes such as:
- The room being too hot or too cold
  - a cooler room is more conducive to sleep
- Poor lighting may cause disorientation or hallucinations (caused by shadows)
- The person may need to urinate and may not be able to find the bathroom
- Changes in the environment can cause disorientation and confusion
- Changes in routine can cause problems sleeping

Things to try:
- Keep the environment as consistent as possible – consistent bedtimes and bedtime rituals
- Check whether the person is too hot or too cold, since dementia can affect a person's internal thermostat
- Shadows, glare or poor lighting may contribute to agitation and hallucinations, so provide nightlights to diminish shadows
- Nightlights may help cut down on confusion at night and may assist the person to find the bathroom
- Make sure the bed and bedroom are comfortable and familiar
  - Familiar objects may help to orient a confused person
- Avoid having daytime clothing in view at night, as this may cause confusion and make the person think it is time to get up
- Make sure that the person is getting adequate exercise; try taking walks each day to use pent-up energy
- If the person is overly tired, consider allowing short naps during the daytime hours

Medications for sleep changes

In some cases, when sleep hygiene and non-drug approaches fail to work or the sleep changes are accompanied by declining health and/or disruptive night-time behaviors, medications may be necessary. Experts recommend that medication treatment follows geriatric prescribing guidelines:

'begin low and go slow' – i.e., use the smallest effective dose possible, give the medication an adequate amount of time to work, increase a medication only when necessary and increase only in small increments, and only use the medication when necessary – weaning and removing it when possible. There are risks associated with the use of medications for sleep problems in older individuals, including an increased risk for falls and fractures. And in those who are cognitively impaired, there is an increased risk of worsening confusion and agitation, which can lead to a decline in the person's ability to perform the activities of daily living. If sleep medications are used, try not to use them on a long term basis and attempt to discontinue them after a regular sleep pattern has been established; also see recommendations in Chapter 8 on Confusion (Alzheimer's Association – Treatment for Sleep, 2010). The type of medication prescribed is often influenced by the behaviors that may accompany the sleep changes.

Types of medications used to treat sleep problems

There are many medications elders may obtain without a prescription which are utilized to manage insomnia as well as several prescription medications. Older individuals should use any medication for insomnia with extreme caution due to the increased risks for causing more falls and injury in these individuals. Use insomnia agents only when necessary and stop using insomnia medications when able to sleep better. If a medication is used on a routine basis, some individuals will build up a tolerance to the medication i.e. if the medication is used continuously (every night), the medication does not seem to work as well as it did when the individual initially started taking the medication. This may cause the person to require higher doses of the medication in order to obtain the desired effect of sleep.

Table 3-3. *Sleeping Medications*

Nonbenzodiazepines
- eszopiclone (Lunesta) — 1, 2, or 3 mg at bedtime only as needed
- zaleplon (Sonata) — 5, 10, or 20 mg at bedtime only as needed
- zolpidem (Ambien) — 5 to10 mg at bedtime only as needed

Benzodiazepines can be a hazard in elders due to potential for falls, worsening of confusion, delusions, and hallucinations as well as potentially increasing agitation

- temazepam (Restoril) — 7.5 to 15mg at bedtime only as needed
- triazolam (Halcion) — 0.125mg to 0.25mg at bedtime only as needed

Melatonin receptor agonists
- ramelteon (Rozerem) — 8 mg at bedtime only as needed

Antihistamines are commonly found in over-the-counter sleeping medication (no prescription necessary to obtain). They are dangerous in older individuals because they can cause worsening of confusion, delusions, hallucinations, and increase the incidence of falls – use cautiously

- diphenhydramine (Benadryl) — 12.5 to 25 mg at bedtime only as needed
- hydroxizine (Atarax) — 12.5 to 25 mg at bedtime only as needed
- meclizine (Antivert) — 12.5 to 25 mg at bedtime only as needed

Melatonin is a naturally-occurring hormone, but it can also be made synthetically and taken as a supplement. It can cause drowsiness and lower body temperature to assist in sleeping. Caution should be used, since it can increase a person's risks for developing blood clotting abnormalities (particularly if the person is also taking warfarin), increased risk of seizure, and disorientation with overdose

- Melatonin — 5 mg at bedtime as needed

(Fragoso & Gill, 2007; Senior Journal, 2006; Mayhew, 2001; Monthly Prescribing Reference (MPR), 2010; Sleepdex, 2010)

Chapter 3 References

Alzheimer's Association. (2010). Treatment for Sleep. Retrieved March 25, 2011, from http://www.alz.org/alzheimers_disease_10429.asp

Better Health Channel. (2010). Dementia and sleeping problems. Retrieved April 17, 2010, from http://www.betterhealth.vic.gov.au/bhcv2/bhcarticles.nsf/pages/Dementia_and_sleeping_problems

Black, E. (2010). Diabetes and Insomnia. Quality Health. Retrieved April 18, 2010, from http://www.qualityhealth.com/diabetes-articles/diabetes-insomnia

Brannon, G., Vij, S., & Gentili, A. (2009). Sleep Disorder, Geriatric. eMedicine from WebMD. Retrieved April 17, 2010, from http://emedicine.medscape.com/article/292498-overview

Chen, J. (2006). To Sleep, Perchance to Dream: An Update on Sleep Disorders. Medscape Pharmacists-Online journal. Retrieved March 24, 2011, from http://www.medscape.com/viewarticle/549682

Fragoso, C., & Gill, T. (2007). Sleep Complaints in Community-Living Older Persons: A Multifactorial Geriatric Syndrome. *Journal of the American Geriatric Society*. 55(11); 1853-1866

Fulcher, K., & White, P. (2000). Strength and physiological response to exercise in patients with chronic fatigue syndrome. *Journal of Neurology, Neurosurgery & Psychiatry 2000*; 69:302-307

Health Guide. (2010). Effects Of Insomnia The Health Problems A Lack Of Sleep Can Cause. Retrieved April 18, 2010, from http://www.fqwz.com/2010/03/health-guide-effects-of-insomnia-the-health-problems-a-lack-of-sleep-can-cause

Kalapatapu, R. & Schimming, C. (2009). Update on neuropsychiatric symptoms of dementia: Antipsychotic use. *Geriatrics*. 64 (5). 10-18.

Mayhew, M. (2001). How should I manage insomnia in the Elderly? Medscape for Nurses. Retrieved April 18, 2010, from http://www.medscape.com/viewarticle/413367

Medical News Today. (2008). Insomnia linked to Hypertension. Retrieved April 18, 2010, from http://www.medicalnewstoday.com/articles/112213.php

Monthly Prescribing Reference (MPR). (2010). Haymarket Media: New York, NY.

Rose, K. & Lorenz, R. (2010). Sleep disturbances in dementia. *Journal of Gerontological Nursing*. 36(5). 9-14.

Senior Journal. (2006) Beers Criteria for mediations to avoid in the elderly. Retrieved October 14, 2006, from http://seniorjournal.com/NEWS/Eldercare/3-12-08Beers.htm

Sleep Disorders (2010). What Causes REM Sleep Behavior Disorder? Retrieved April 18, 2010, from http://apneasleepdisorders.com/what-causes-rem-sleep-behavior-disorder

Sleepdex. (2010). Sleep aides for seniors. Retrieved April 18, 2010, from http://www.sleepdex.org/senior-meds.htm

Zec, & Burkett, (2008). Non-pharmacological and pharmacological treatment of the cognitive and behavioral symptoms of Alzheimer's disease. *Journal of NeuroRehabilitation*. (23). 425-438.

Chapter 4

Pain

Pain may be acute, but it is often chronic in many older adults for a variety of reasons, and can lead to a diminished quality of life. It is often caused by arthritis and can lead to immobility and falls in elders. Pain management includes paying special attention to activity, positioning, and pharmacological management. Strategies to manage pain in elders will be presented with a focus on precautions for the use of medications in elders. Geriatric dosages are encouraged, as well as appropriate monitoring of laboratory values, to prevent other complications..

Pain is an unpleasant sensation which is both a sensory and emotional experience associated with an actual or potential tissue injury. It is whatever the person says it is and is more than a feeling or a change in the nervous system; it is also reflective of the patient's past experiences with pain, as well as the meaning the individual believes the pain signifies. Pain can be present even when a person cannot communicate it.

Acute pain begins suddenly and can be sharp in quality. It serves as a warning of a problem, such as a disease or a threat to the body. It may be mild and last only a short period of time – minutes or hours – or it may be severe and last for an extended period of time – weeks or months. In most cases, acute pain usually disappears when the underlying cause has been treated or the problem has resolved. Any acute pain which is not resolved may lead to chronic pain.

Chronic pain is pain lasting longer than one month or pain that continues despite the fact that the cause of pain has resolved or an injury has healed. It can cause muscle tension, limited mobility, fatigue, and changes in appetite as well as sleep. Other effects can include depression, anxiety, and fear of re-injury, which can affect a person's daily life.

Types of Pain

Muscle pain such as fibromyalgia and myofascial pain

Inflammatory pain is commonly associated with acute pain such as postoperative site and injury

Chronic inflammatory pain includes arthritis, fibromyalgia, inflammatory bowel syndrome

Mechanical pain created by pressure or stretching and can result in complications such as a fracture or dislocation as well as compression of tissue by bony structures, or pressure on skin

Psychological pain includes depression, anxiety, personality disorders, somatization, and post-traumatic stress.

Other types of pain Headaches, Low back pain, Cancer pain, Shingles pain, and Neurogenic pain (pain resulting from damage to nerves)

Table 4-1. *Types of Arthritis*		
Arthritis is a chronic problem many elders experience and can lead to pain, disability, and reduced quality of life. The key is to stay active i.e. keep moving and manage pain through medication management. There are three types of arthritis afflicting over half of the elderly population.		
Rheumatoid Arthritis	**Osteoarthritis**	**Gouty Arthritis**
CAUSE An autoimmune disorder which affects the lining of a person's joints, causing pain, swelling, and problems with movement. It can eventually result in bone erosion and joint deformity	Osteoarthritis is also referred to as degenerative joint disease and is the most common form of arthritis in older individuals. It occurs when cartilage in the joints wears down over time.	An accumulation in joints of uric acid or urate crystals, causing inflammation and intense pain. An acute flare-up is referred to as a gout attack. Normally, the body produces uric acid when it breaks down purines, which are substances that are found naturally in the body as well as in certain foods. Urate crystals can form when a person has high levels of uric acid in the blood. Urate crystals can accumulate in the joint and cause pain.

(CONTINUED)

Table 4-1. Types of Arthritis (CONTINUED)

	Rheumatoid Arthritis	Osteoarthritis	Gouty Arthritis
SYMPTOMS	• Joint pain • Joint swelling • Joints that are tender to the touch • Red and puffy hands • Firm bumps of tissue under the skin on the arms and hands, also referred to as rheumatoid nodules • Fatigue • Morning stiffness that may last for hours	• Symptoms progressively worsen over time • Joint pain is worse during or after movement • Tenderness of joint with palpation or pressing on joint • Loss of flexibility • Grating sensation with joint movement, also referred to as crepitus	• A gout flare-up: an acute attack of pain in a joint – commonly affects the great toe • Pain in the joint may begin suddenly then linger for weeks • Pain in joints commonly moves to a different joint
TYPICAL PRESENTATION	• Stiffness and pain worse in the morning – may last up to 2 hours after rising or stiffness and pain after periods of inactivity	• Pain in joint is worse during or after activity or use of the joint	• Redness, swelling, and warmth of the affected joint • Movement irritates or worsens the symptoms
DIAGNOSING	• Physical Examination • X-rays • Blood test: Elevated Sed Rate (ESR)	• Physical Examination • X-rays • Blood test: Normal Sed Rate (ESR)	• Physical Examination • X-rays • Blood tests to assess uric acid levels – possibly an elevated Uric Acid level • Joint aspiration to assess for presence of urate crystals

(CONTINUED)

	Rheumatoid Arthritis	Osteoarthritis	Gouty Arthritis
MEDICATION MANAGEMENT	• Anti-inflammatory Nonsteroidal Drugs (NSAIDS) such as ibuprofen, naproxen, or other prescription medications • Stronger pain medications (refer to Pain Medication Table) • Steroid medications • Anti-rheumatic medications • Immunosuppressant medications • Fish oil • Other prescription medications	• Acetaminophen • NSAIDS such as ibuprofen, naproxen, or other prescription medications • Stronger pain medications (refer to Pain Medication Table) • Steroid medications – injections or oral therapy	• Anti-inflammatory Nonsteroidal Drugs (NSAIDS) such as ibuprofen, naproxen, or other prescription medications, including colchicine and indomethacin • Steroid medications
LIFESTYLE MANAGEMENT	• Use ice alternating with heat therapy • Exercise to stretch and strengthen as well as maintain or improve balance • Relaxation techniques • Gait and Balance assessment and gait training with use of assistive devices, if necessary	• Use heat therapy • Non-stressful exercises • Relaxation techniques • Balance assessment and gait training with use of assistive devices, if necessary	• Rest when a joint is inflamed • Increase fluid intake • Avoid alcohol • Eat only a moderate amount of protein such as limiting daily intake of meat, fish and poultry to 4 to 6 ounces • Consider alternative management: Coffee, Vitamin C 500 mg daily, & increasing intake of blackberries, blueberries, purple grapes and raspberries OR Black Cherry Pills 1000mg daily

Pain is the 5th Vital Sign

An individual's perception of pain differs from one person to the next. Pain is assessed based on several factors: self-report from the individual, observation of physical symptoms such as guarding and mobility, and behavioral symptoms. An individual's perception of pain is the most important and reliable factor to evaluate. Pain can be verbalized or rated on a scale from *no pain at all* to *the worst pain someone has ever experienced.* 0 or 1 usually is equivalent to *No Pain* and the higher number is the most intense pain a person has experienced.

Pain Characteristics

Assess characteristics and causes of pain and how much is known about the pain, including the frequency or chronicity of pain. Evaluate for any precipitating and alleviating factors. Assessment of any current and previous pain management approaches is essential to establish an appropriate plan of care or management.

Sometimes, it is necessary to treat pain before all relevant information has been gathered or the cause has been sought or identified. BUT caution must be used not to mask the cause of the pain, due to the potential problem of missing an acute problem in an elder. Treatment should be aimed at comfort, tolerability, and preventing complications. Management should be targeted to the most likely source of pain, but should still follow systematic approach to treatment beginning with comfort measures, light pain medications and then, if necessary, stronger medications or alternative treatments.

Pain assessment and proper diagnosis depends on the use of accurate historical and clinical information, along with physical evidence derived from an appropriate direct examination. Consider additional examinations by the primary care provider and possibly specialists/consultations when the goal remains to identify causes and develop an appropriate treatment plan.

PAIN MANAGEMENT

Pain is one of the most difficult issues to assess and manage in elders. It is often hard to determine the level of pain a person is experiencing, since every individual will feel pain differently and it may be difficult to correlate objective findings with a particular condition. No known interventions, whether medication or non-pharmacologic, are effective for every type of pain in every individual. Commonly, medications are used to manage pain, but all medications (including analgesics) carry substantial risks and may be highly problematic (including causing death) when not used cautiously in older individuals (AMDA, 2002).

The key principles of pain management are similar in management of both acute pain and chronic pain. It is always important to identify the cause of pain and attempt to remove the cause, if possible. Pain may predispose an individual to complications, including problems with mobility, getting around, and remaining independent. Other problems to which pain can contribute include depression, social isolation, difficulty in eating, and sleep problems. In individuals with cognitive impairment or problems communicating their needs, pain may not be readily reported by the individual or described appropriately, so it may not addressed in developing a plan of care for that person. Signs and symptoms that suggest a person is experiencing pain include grimacing, restlessness, increased agitation, resisting care, or crying. It is important to try to identify nonspecific symptoms of pain and attempt to comfort the person, as well as alleviate the pain.

MANAGING PAIN – Lifestyle Modifications

Reduce stress – avoid or limit activity which causes pain, avoid overexertion and emotional stress. Allow for relaxation. AND encourage a person to learn how to say 'no' without guilt.

Get enough sleep – allot enough time for sleep, practice good sleep habits by going to bed and getting up at the same time each day, as well as limiting daytime napping.

Exercise regularly to maintain or develop balance, strength, and stamina. If not very active, start slowly and build up gradually. Many older individuals find exercises such as walking, swimming, bicycling and water aerobics to be beneficial. Stretching, good posture and relaxation exercises also assist in diminishing pain intensity.

Pace lifestyle – keep activity on an even level. If a person does too much on good days, they may have more bad days.

Maintain a healthy lifestyle – eating a balanced diet, drinking plenty of water, limiting caffeine intake, stopping smoking, getting an adequate amount of rest, and exercising regularly.

Maintain an ideal weight-if overweight – lose weight since every pound a person is overweight causes increased stress on knees by three to five pounds during walking. A ten pound weight loss can improve a person's health since it will alleviate stress on knee joints by 30 to 50 pounds (Eustice, 2006).

Chronic Pain

Chronic pain is experienced by many elders and may interfere with normal functioning as well as diminish a person's quality of life. A significant number of older individuals do not receive adequate pain management due to four significant factors: (1) lack of proper pain assessment; (2) potential risks of pharmacotherapy in the elderly person; (3) misconceptions regarding both the efficacy of nonpharmacological pain management strategies; and (4) misconceptions that pain is acceptable in an older person and is a normal expectation with aging. In care of older adults, practitioners must be judicious in managing pain in order to allow elders to live up to their full functional abilities as well as their optimal potential.

Pain is a complex phenomenon caused by sensory stimuli or neuropathological mechanisms. Acute pain is a sign of real or impending tissue damage and usually disappears with healing. It can be a normal predicted physiologic response and occurs for a short duration. Persistent pain continues for a prolonged period of time and may or may not be associated with a disease process. In the medical literature, the terms "persistent pain" and "chronic pain" are often used interchangeably (AGS, 2010). Chronic pain can be defined by multiple different time frames (generally from 6 weeks to 3 months after the onset of symptoms). It has also been defined as pain that persists for at least 30 days beyond the expected course of an illness. Chronic pain is a condition that adversely affects the patient's well being, level of function and quality of life (Sangl, 2007).

	Table 4-2. *Initial Evaluation for Chronic Pain*
History	1. Determine the cause of the pain, the type of pain, and all diagnoses
	2. Determine if there was a specific incident that caused or triggered the onset of pain or if the pain had a slow onset
	3. Determine the severity and specific location of the pain (including if the pain is radiating)
	4. Determine if the pain is localized at one site or if it became more multifocal/generalized

	5. Determine characteristics of the pain:
	a. Quality of pain – descriptions may include aching, dull, sharp, burning, electric, dysesthesia, paresthesias, and/or neuralgia
	b. Is it acute or chronic; continuous or intermittent; the same pain or changing in character
	c. Any associated neurological factors
	  o weakness
	  o numbness
	  o balance problems
	d. Any factors that exacerbate or relieve the pain
	e. Any effect of activity, body position, and mobility to relieve or exacerbate the pain
	f. Any effect of stress or fatigue

	6. Determine what previous evaluations or tests have been done
	7. Determine the effect of previous treatment, including medications, lifestyle, or exercise
	8. Assess the ability of the individual to perform functions such as walking, lifting, sitting, standing, and reclining
	9. Assess for evidence of substance abuse in the patient, in the past or currently – including alcohol, smoking, or illicit drugs. Assess for any history of over-use or abuse of prescription and/or over-the-counter pain medications
	10. Examine for evidence of concordant depression, anxiety, other mood disturbance, sleep disturbance, or eating disturbance

(AGS, 2010; Wikipedia, 2010)

Recognizing pain in cognitively-impaired elders

Recognition of pain in cognitively-impaired elders is much more difficult. Many of these elders have pain on a chronic basis and are unable to communicate this appropriately, especially if they have a history of arthritis or there are apparent arthritic deformities. Observations should be made during movement or palpation of a suspected area of pain, when an elder is more likely to perceive pain and cry out. Other indicators may include poor appetite, depressive symptoms, sleep problems, change of function, agitated behavior, refusal of care, moans, groans, or crying. Observe the resident for three to five minutes, paying particular attention to 'unusual' behaviors.

Table 4-3. *Pain Assessment in Cognitively-Impaired Individuals*	
Do	**Don't Do**
• Use an instrument with simple language • Use simple words to describe pain ('aching', 'hurting') • Ask 'yes/no' questions o Be cautious with individuals who answer yes or no to all questions • Listen for clues in speech, even if speech is fragmented • Palpate areas thought to be painful while asking questions • Assess pain following or during movement • Attempt to assess pain in individual with poor appetite, depressive symptoms, sleep problems, changes of function, agitated behavior, or those who refuse care • Observe for nonverbal symptoms such as furrowed brows, grimaces, groans, and crying out during movement	• Don't use the verbal 1 to 10 scale; it may be too complex • Don't discount behaviors as part of dementia • Don't use small-print instruments • Don't interrupt attempts at responses • Don't assume that anti-anxiety medications will relieve pain • Don't forget to ask family members about previous pain complaints of the person • Don't overlook the possibility of discomfort due to urinary tract infections, constipation, or compression fractures in frail elders • Don't assume that persons with dementia don't experience pain

Source: Feldt KS, Improving assessment and treatment of pain in cognitively impaired nursing home residents. Annals of Long-Term Care 2000;8 (9): 36-42.

General Treatment for Pain Management
A general plan for managing pain in elders includes:

1. Develop a plan of care that addresses the elder's personal goals, sleep, physical activity, stress management, and recommendations to improve pain control
2. Include the elder in the treatment plan
3. Incorporate environmental adaptation to decrease pain occurrence, as well as develop a routine to prevent fatigue
4. Consider the use of a cognitive behavioral program, when indicated

MANAGEMENT OF CHRONIC PAIN

It may be difficult to make chronic pain go away completely, but it can be lessened and made tolerable so that an elder has a better quality of life. Medication management cannot be used alone and must be used in conjunction with behavioral and environmental strategies. Environment is an important factor to consider; having an elder go to a quiet place may make it easier for the person to tolerate pain. Avoiding bright lights or loud, noisy places can also help control pain. Making sure an environment is not too hot or too cold may assist to decrease pain – consider hot and/or cold packs to help minimize pain. Remember that a long warm bath may help calm an individual and let their muscles relax. Laughter may help a person take deep breaths – it lowers blood pressure and may cause a person's brain to create endorphins, which will decrease pain perception. Laughter can help change a person's mood, encourages relaxation and allows a person to let go of stress, anger, fear, depression, and hopelessness. Massage is another technique used to manage pain and assist in relaxation. Massage can be even more effective if you also use guided imagery, breathing exercises, or music accompaniment. Physical therapy can be helpful with pain caused by immobility and stiffness. Stretching muscles and making them stronger around the area of pain can help diminish the pain. Other considerations include aromatherapy, acupuncture, hypnosis, spinal cord stimulation, transcutaneous electrical nerve stimulation (TENS), and touch energy therapies (Drugs.com, 2010).

How is pain treated? The goal of therapy is to relieve pain and improve quality of life for an older person. Many pain medications work by blocking pain signals going to the brain or by changing how the brain interprets pain signals. When using medications to manage pain, it is recommended to use the least amount of medications possible to manage the pain; this will help to avoid adverse effects of the treatment.

Pain Medication Classifications

Non-narcotic analgesics: These work by changing the way the body senses pain and by cooling the body. Non-narcotic analgesics are used to relieve mild to moderate pain from headaches, muscle aches, colds, and fever

- Acetaminophen – caution: no more than 4000mg/24hours
  REMEMBER – Many other pain medications contain Acetaminophen
- Tramadol (Ultram) 50 mg every 6 hours as needed for pain

Non-steroidal anti-inflammatory drugs: This family of medicine, also called NSAIDs, helps decrease pain and inflammation (swelling). Some NSAIDs may also be used to decrease a high body temperature or fever

- Celecoxib (Celebrex) 200 mg once a day
- Ibuprofen (Motrin, Advil) 50 to 100 mg twice a day
- Indomethacin (Indocin) 25 to 50 mg three or four times a day-Also treats gout *if allergic to aspirin-avoid taking indocin
- Meloxicam (Mobic) 7.5 to 15mg twice a day
- Naproxen (Naprosyn, Aleve) 250, 375, 500 mg twice a day
- Piroxicam (Feldene) 10 mg twice a day

Narcotic analgesics: Many of these medicines, which include morphine, contain opium. A narcotic analgesic is used for the management of moderate to severe pain. This may be used to control cancer pain and chronic pain, as well as pain after surgery or other procedures.

- Narcotic Analgesics (which can cause hallucinations, falls, and agitation in elders) include Morphine and Dilaudid – if used, use extreme precautions
  o Narcotic Analgesics often used after orthopedic surgery include Lortab, Lorcet, Oxycodone, and Percocet

What other medicines may be given to help pain? Other medications can be used in conjunction with, or in place of, stronger pain medications. Pain caused by infections may be treated with antibiotic or anti-viral medicine. Pain from cancer may be treated with chemotherapy or radiation therapy. Some types of pain are managed with steroids.

Table 4-4. *Alternative Pain Management*
Anti-anxiety medicine: This medicine may be given to decrease anxiety, treat nervousmess and encourage relaxation
Anticonvulsant medicine: Anticonvulsants are usually given to control seizures but have a side effect of calming a person, which may also diminish the pain
Anti-depressants: A symptom of depression can be chronic medical issues, including pain – some antidepressants are indicated for depression and peripheral neuralgia (Cymbalta)
Muscle relaxers: When muscles are relaxed, pain can more easily be controlled and possibly the elder may have less pain
Steroids: This class of medications may be given to decrease inflammation, which is redness, pain, and swelling – CAUTION steroids can cause psychosis in elders

NOTE: Dosing pain medications in elders requires monitoring for changes in level of consciousness, risks for falls, and other problems common in elders.

Pain Management Principles

Some general principles should be followed to manage pain: reassurance, comfortable positioning especially in bed or chair-bound individuals, and a comfortable, supportive environment. Simple measures may bring substantial relief and reduce the need for analgesics, or at least allow lower doses to be used.

Goals of a person-centered approach to developing a plan of care should be based on an individual's preferences, as well as knowledge of the pain's location, characteristics, and causes, as well as the person's condition, prognosis, risk factors, co-morbidities, and existing medication regimen. It is important to establish realistic expectations – is the goal pain relief or pain management? Determine whether underlying causes of pain can be corrected and how long it may take to identify the best plan of care with the fewest side effects and the least risk for complications.

While medications are commonly used to manage pain, all medications (including analgesics) have benefits and risks that may vary; it is important to consider other medications a person is concurrently taking, and the individual's current diagnoses. It is essential to use medications correctly and judiciously while monitoring for complications, which can include falls, aspiration, and sedation. The responsible use of analgesics can be beneficial, but less cautious approaches could lead to serious complications, including death. The World Health Organization (WHO) has recommended a three-tier 'stepladder' approach to pain management. It is important to make individual-specific decisions based on these general guidelines: first – attempt to alleviate the cause of the pain and/or modify a person's activity and environment; next – use over-the-counter (mild) pain medications and lastly, if necessary – use stronger, prescription-strength medications to manage pain.

**GUIDELINES FOR PAIN MANAGEMENT

- Opioid analgesics are appropriate for moderate to severe pain that is not relieved by, or is unlikely to respond to, other categories of analgesics.
- While the judicious use of opioid analgesics is often helpful, this class of medications can cause significant complications in susceptible individuals, including anorexia, hypotension, falling, severe constipation, and lethargy as well as confusion. Some may be problematic when a patient's additional decline or discomfort is more likely due to the treatment than to the underlying illnesses. Preventive measures should be taken to prevent constipation, such as establishing a bowel regimen, for individuals receiving opioid analgesics.
- Consider complementary therapies, such as physical and behavioral treatments, including exercise and heat or cold applications that may be used alone or in combination with appropriate drug regimens to help manage pain.

- Re-evaluate pain and adjust treatment plans as necessary
- It is essential to reassess pain periodically and to assess the effectiveness of the management of pain symptoms. Assessment should include monitoring functional capacity, walking abilities and fall risks, sleep patterns, and participation in usual activities. It is also important to monitor for possible adverse consequences of analgesic medications. Sometimes, analgesics can be decreased in dosages or frequency as well as tapered and discontinued, at other times they should continue for a longer duration, if not indefinitely.
- Evaluate if pain is controlled: key to effective pain management is reviewing and repeating the steps in this guideline as appropriate until the individual's pain is controlled or it is determined that no further improvement is likely.

(Levenson, 2007)

BASICS OF PAIN MANAGEMENT WITH MEDICATIONS IN ELDERS
Managing pain should be prompt with use of oral agents in the following order:
1. Nonopioids (aspirin and acetaminophen) with or without adjuvant analgesics
2. Then, as necessary, mild opioids (codeine) with or without adjuvant analgesics
3. Then strong opioids such as morphine or an equivalent, until the patient is free of pain with or without adjuvant analgesics

(WHO Ladder Guidelines, 2010)

PAIN MANAGEMENT – MEDICATION CONSIDERATIONS
Acetaminophen
- Relieves mild to moderate pain (changing the way the body senses pain) as well as reduces fever
- Dosing greater than 4 gm daily can cause liver damage

Salicylates – Aspirin & Enteric Coated Aspirin
- Decrease pain
- May increase the risk of bleeding (including bleeding in the stomach)

Non-Steroidal Anti-inflammatory Drugs (NSAIDs):
- Reduce the sensation of pain
- At higher doses, they reduce the inflammation that often accompanies and worsens pain
  o Ibuprofen, ketoprofen, & naproxen

Potential Problems:
- **Problems in the digestive tract:** All NSAIDs tend to irritate the stomach's lining and cause digestive upset (heartburn, indigestion, nausea, bloating, diarrhea, and stomach pain), peptic ulcers, and bleeding in the digestive tract (gastrointestinal bleeding). Taking NSAIDs with food and using antacids may help prevent stomach irritation. Proton pump inhibitors (omeprazole – PRILOSEC) or histamine-2 (H2) blockers (famotidine – PEPCID) can also help prevent stomach problems due to NSAIDs.
- **Bleeding problems:** All NSAIDs except coxibs interfere with the clotting tendency of platelets and lead to increased occurrence of bleeding, especially in the digestive tract if they also irritate the stomach's lining.
- **Problems related to retaining fluids:** NSAIDs cause swelling in some people. Regular use of NSAIDs may also increase the risk of developing a kidney disorder and may result in kidney damage and failure.
- **Increased risk of heart and blood vessel disorders:** Recent studies suggest that all NSAIDs (except aspirin) increase the risk of heart attack, stroke, and blood clots in the legs. The risk appears to be higher with higher doses and longer use of the drug. The risk is also higher with some NSAIDs than with others. These problems may be related directly to the drug's effect on clotting or indirectly to a small but persistent increase in blood pressure caused by the drug.

Coxibs (COX-2 Inhibitors): Coxibs, such as celecoxib (Celebrex), differ from other NSAIDs. Other NSAIDs block two enzymes:
- COX-1, which is involved in the production of prostaglandins that protect the stomach and play a crucial role in blood clotting
- COX-2, which is involved in the production of prostaglandins that promote inflammation
- Potential problems: Coxibs (COX-2 inhibitors) are less likely to irritate the stomach and cause bleeding than other NSAIDs. However, if people are taking a coxib and aspirin concurrently, these problems are just as likely.

Opioid Agents
- Decrease perception of pain and an individual's reaction to pain, as well as increase the pain tolerance
- Potential problems: sedation, respiratory depression, constipation, confusion, agitation, falls, and death in elders

(Merck Manual-Pain Management, 2010)

More Aggressive Pain Management may involve the use of opioid analgesics, also referred to as narcotics, which are the most powerful analgesics available. They are often used in the treatment of severe acute pain and chronic pain due to cancer and other serious disorders. Opioids are effective in controlling pain because they are chemically related to morphine (a natural substance extracted from poppies, but which can also be manufactured in a laboratory). The administration of an opioid is begun with a low dose and then increased gradually until the pain is relieved or the opioid's side effects cannot be tolerated. Side effects of opioid drugs are more likely to occur in people with certain conditions, such as kidney failure, liver disease, chronic obstructive pulmonary disease (COPD), dementia, or another brain disorder. POTENTIAL PROBLEMS, including drowsiness, constipation, nausea, vomiting, and itching, are common when opioids are started (Merck Manual-Pain Management, 2010)

Pain Management Medications in Older Adults

Table 4-5. *Non-Opioid Medications*		
Medication	**Geriatric Dosing Recommendations**	**Precautions**
acetaminophen (Tylenol)	325-500 mg every 4-6 hours as needed (occasionally for pain 500-1000mg every 4-6 hours)	If liver disease – dosing may be lower No more than 4000 mg/24 hours or can cause liver damage
celecoxib (Celebrex)	100-200 mg daily (usually routinely given daily)	High doses can cause problems with gastrointestinal irritation and worsen cardiovascular disease IF on aspirin, consider using a gastrointestinal protectant
naproxen sodium (Naprosyn)	220 mg every 12 hours as needed for pain	Studies have indicated that this agent has less cardiovascular effects than other agents in this class
ibuprofen (Motrin)	200 mg every 8 hours as needed for pain	Possible interaction with aspirin: it has been suggested that ibuprofen potentially interferes with the cardioprotective benefits of aspirin
diclofenac sodium (Voltaren)	50 mg twice a day or 75 mg extended release formulation-once a day	Potential worsening of cardiovascular disease – similar to Non-steroidal anti-inflammatory agents (NSAIDS)
diclofenac/ misoprostol (Arthrotec)	50 mg or 75 mg twice a day	Potential worsening of cardiovascular disease and high risk of developing NSAID-induced gastric and duodenal ulcers and their complications
etodolac (Lodine)	200-400 mg every 6 to 8 hours – do not exceed 1200 mg/day	Potential worsening of cardiovascular disease – similar to Non-steroidal anti-inflammatory agents (NSAIDS)
indomethacin (Indocin)	25 mg dose given 2-3 times/day	May cause GI upset, bleeding, ulceration, perforation; take with food or milk to minimize GI upset

(CONTINUED)

Table 4-5. *Non-Opioid Medications (CONTINUED)*

Medication	Geriatric Dosing Recommendations	Precautions
nabumentone (Relafen)	1 mg daily	This agent has a relatively long half-life (stays in system for over 5 days) and has minimal blood thinning properties
ketorolac (Toradol)	Renal insufficiency or weight < 50 kg: 10 mg every 4-6 hours as needed for pain May be given injectable (IM) 15-30 mg every 6 hours as needed for pain (do not exceed 60mg/24hours) May also be given intravenously (IV) 15mg every 6 hours as needed for pain. *If the person has renal disease or weighs less than 100 lbs-use lower dosages	Not normally recommended in older individuals due to gastrointestinal and cardiovascular effects. Elders have increased occurrence of bleeding in the stomach/gastrointestinal tract, ulceration, and perforation Also if decreased Creatinine clearance – do not exceed 60 mg/day.
piroxicam (Feldene)	10-20 mg once or twice a day	Potential worsening of cardiovascular disease and high risk of developing NSAID-induced gastric and duodenal ulcers and their complications
sulindac (Clinoril)	150-200 mg twice daily or 300 mg once daily (not to exceed 400 mg/day)	Potential worsening of cardiovascular disease and high risk of developing NSAID-induced gastric and duodenal ulcers and their complications Not recommended for use in incapacitated elders

Table 4-6. *Opioid Medications*		
Medication	**Geriatric Dosing Recommendations**	**Precautions**
codeine (Tylenol #3, Tylenol #4, Codimal PH, any cough medication with codine)	10 to 15 mg every 6 hours as needed for pain	A weak narcotic pain medication and cough suppressant. May be habit forming and is not commonly used to manage chronic pain in elders.
hydrocodone (Lorcet, Lortab, Norco, Vicoden, Vicoprofen)	2.5 to 5mg every 4-6 hours as needed for acute pain or breakthrough pain in chronic pain management (maximum dose is 60 mg/day)	Caution should be used in hydrocodone agents which also have acetaminophen – caution not to take more than the maximum of 4000 mg/day of acetaminophen which can cause liver damage. These agents have a risk of increasing the incidence of orthostatic hypotension, falls, and confusion in certain elders.
oxycodone (Oxycontin, Percocet, Percodan, Tylox, Combunox)	5-10mg every 12 hours as needed for acute pain or breakthrough pain in chronic pain management	Caution should be used in hydrocodone agents which also have acetaminophen – watching not to reach the maximum 4000 mg/day of acetaminophen which can cause liver damage. These agents have a risk of increasing the incidence of orthostatic hypotension, falls, and confusion in certain elders.
morphine immediate release forms: (MSRI, Roxanol)	2.5-10 mg every 4 hours as needed for pain	Immediate release forms available in pill or liquid formulation.
extended release forms: (Avinza, Kadian, MS Contin, Oramorph SR) **transdermal formulation: (Duramorph)**	15 mg every 8-12 hours as needed or routinely dosed in chronic pain management	*All Morphine agents can cause orthostatic hypotension, falls, confusion, hallucination, and agitation in certain elders. MORPHINE is reserved for pain which is not managed with other agents.

(CONTINUED)

Table 4-6. *Opioid Medications (CONTINUED)*

Medication	Geriatric Dosing Recommendations	Precautions
hydromorphine (Dilaudid, Hydrostat)	1-2 mg every 3-4 hours as needed for pain management	Same potential problems as Morphine – see above.
methadone (Dolophine)		Not recommended as a first line agent and should only be prescribed by practitioners who are expert at pain management.
oxymorphone: immediate release (Opana IR)	5 mg every 6 hours as needed for pain management	Same potential problems as Morphine – see above. Potential interactions with foods and alcohol.
tramadol (Ultram) *non-narcotic but a synthetic opioid analgesic	50 mg every 6 hours as needed for pain (not to exceed 400 mg/day; geriatric recommendations 200 mg/day)	Potential interactions with many medications, a medication interaction should be assessed prior to use; can cause confusion, sedation, agitation, and falls in elders.
transdermal fentanyl (Duragesic patches)	12-25 mcg/hour-patch applied once every 72 hours (3 days) may be used in higher doses up to 100mcg/hour patches	Same potential problems as Morphine – see above. The patch takes 18 to 24 hours to reach pain control levels and other agents may be needed until the patch reaches a good blood level for pain management. Patch may not be cut or dosing will not be delivered over the entire 72 hours.

	Table 4-7. *Alternative Management/Other Therapies for Pain Management in Older Adults*	
These agents are not indicated for pain management but are being used based on expert suggestions and evidenced-based practices.		
Medication	**Geriatric Dosing Recommendations**	**Precautions**
duloxetine (Cymbalta)	30-60 mg daily	It is indicated as an antidepressant and indicated to manage fibromyalgia and neuropathic pain. There are potential adverse effects in elders, including interactions with other medications, cardiovascular effects (affecting blood pressure), increased confusion or agitation, dizziness, and worsening of short-term memory.
venlafexine (Effexor)	37.5-75 mg daily	Indicated as an antidepressant. Potential to increase blood pressure and heart-rate.
carbamazepine (Tegretol)	100 mg daily	Indicated as an anti-convulsant. Monitor for sedation, ataxia, and edema.
pregabalin (*Lyrica) *controlled substance	50-100 mg daily at bedtime	Monitor for sedation, ataxia, and edema.
gabapentin (Neurontin)	100 mg daily at bedtime Or 100-300 mg twice a day or three times a day	Indicated as an anti-convulsant. Monitor for sedation, ataxia, and edema.
lamotrigine (Lamictal)	25 mg daily at bedtime	Indicated as an anti-convulsant. Monitor for sedation, ataxia, confusion, and memory problems. In rare cases – Stevens Johnson Syndrome (skin sloughing).

(CONTINUED)

Table 4-7. *Alternative Management/Other Therapies for Pain Management in Older Adults*
(CONTINUED)

Medication	Geriatric Dosing Recommendations	Precautions
corticosteroids (Prednisone, Decadron, Depomedrol, Deltasone, Medrol dose pack, Pred-Pack, Liquipred, Orasone)	If using prednisone – start low doses, wean off when possible If using higher doses – 10-20 mg daily and wean slowly over 1 to 2 weeks	Steroids are indicated for management of inflammation as well as shingles and thus the pain also decreases. Steroids have potential side effects including decreasing immunity or resistance to infection, can cause thinning of bones and increase risks of fractures, can cause increased glucose levels in diabetics, and cause increased confusion, agitation, and insomnia in certain older adults.
lidocaine topical (Lidoderm)	1-3 patches every 12 hours as needed for pain *patch should be removed and do not immediately apply new patch – individual needs 1-3 hours of patch free time to improve pain management **place patch directly over the site of pain for the best results	Potential for rash or irritation at the site of the patch.
baclofen (Lioresal)	5 mg every 8 hours as needed	Indicated for management of muscle spasms. Potential problems include muscle weakness, inability to empty bladder or possible urinary incontinence, increased confusion, and sedation.
tizanidine (Zanaflex)	2 mg every 8 hours as needed	Indicated to manage muscle spasms. Has the same cautions/ problems as Baclofen – (see above).
lorazepam (Ativan)	1-2 mg every 8 hours as needed	Indicated to manage anxiety. Occasionally used to relax an older person to diminish pain. Potential problems include orthostatic hypotension, falls, sedation, confusion, and memory impairment in certain older adults.

(Pain Management Guideline, 2009)

Pain Medication Addiction and Misuse in Elders

Seniors account for the consumption of approximately one quarter of all the prescription drugs that are sold in the United States, and that number continues to rise every year (Gonzalez, 2009). Many elders take medications to manage chronic pain, which increases the risks of addiction and misuse. The likelihood of this is especially great when pain medications are prescribed to an elderly person on a routine basis. In regulating chronic pain, it is very common for an individual to believe increasing the dose or frequency will alleviate the pain better. If this continues for an extended period of time, a person may develop a physical dependency, and sometimes a psychological addiction as well as complications from the use of too many medications. The best plan for preventing this problem (or identifying there is a problem) is monitoring pain medication usage.

As people age, their bodies go through a variety of physiological changes that alter the way they are able to metabolize or process medications. Metabolism actually slows down as an individual gets older – the liver is not as efficient in processing and eliminating medications and the kidneys become smaller in size and not as efficient in filtering medications out of a person's system, and there is a greater chance of gastrointestinal bleeding. All of these factors can play a critical role in determining whether a particular drug is safe for an elderly person, as well as in evaluating chronic use of medications to identify problems. An older person is at a greater risk for experiencing side effects from medications due to the slower processing of medications through their system; this can lead to increased levels of medications circulating in their bloodstream. Even something as basic as acetaminophen (Tylenol®) can produce problems more rapidly than it might in a younger adult due to toxic effects (Gonzalez, 2009).

If there is suspicion that an elderly person is addicted to prescription drugs that are not necessary, or the medications are being misused and are causing problems (falls, confusion, decline in function, etc.), the safest way to manage the issue is to seek assistance from a healthcare professional – making them aware of the suspected problems and asking for advice.

REMEMBER: Many elders are vulnerable to pain due to the various illnesses they are prone to developing. Practitioners are obligated to manage pain in elders to improve quality of life as well as to maintain/ improve function and independence. Pain management should take into consideration many strategies, including behavioral management, environmental manipulation, and medication use. Steps to managing pain include assessment – identifying the type/cause of pain; starting with mild medications – at low doses, allowing an adequate amount of time for efficacy, increasing the dose as needed, changing the medication if necessary, and/or adding adjunct medication(s) to manage pain. Re-assess pain management to determine the effectiveness of treatment, tolerability, possible adverse effects, and achieving the goals of the patient – pain tolerance or pain eradication.

Pain

Chapter 4 References

AGS Clinical Practice Guideline: Pharmacological Management of Persistent Pain in Older Persons: Executive summary. Retrieved December 26, 2010, from http://www.americangeriatrics.org/health_care_professionals/clinical_practice/clinical_guidelines_recommendations/persistent_pain_executive_summary

AMDA (2002). AMDA's Clinical Practice Guideline on Pain Management in the Long Term Care Setting.

Clinicans Ultimate Reference (2010). Retrieved December 26, 2010, from http://www.globalrph.com/nsaids.htm

Drugs.com (2010). Non-pharmacological Pain Management Therapies for Adults. Retrieved December 26, 2010, from http://www.drugs.com/cg/non-pharmacological-pain-management-therapies-for-adults.html

Eustice, C. (2009). Extra Pounds increase Arthritis Pain. About.com. Retrieved July 31, 2011, from http://arthritis.about.com/cs/diet/a/extrapounds.htm

Feldt, K., (2000) Improving assessment and treatment of pain in cognitively impaired nursing home residents. *Annals of Long-Term Care*; 8 (9): 36-42

Ferris, M. (2008). Pain in the Cognitively Impaired Elderly: Guidance for Clinicians. Medscape Nurses. Retrieved December 26, 2010, from http://www.medscape.com/viewarticle/573642_3

Gonzalez, J. (2009). Pain medication and the Elderly. Retrieved December 17, 2010, from http://www.everythingaddiction.com/populations/elderly/pain-meds-elderly

Levenson, S. (2007). Pain Needs to Be Managed One Step at a Time. Caring for the Ages. 8(5). pp 14-15.

Merck Manual for Geriatrics (2010). Pain Management. Retrieved December 26, 2010, from http://www.merckmanuals.com/professional/search.html?qt=pain+manegement&qp=%2Bsite%3Awww%2Emerckmanuals%2Ecom+%2Burl%3A%2Fprofessional+%2Durl%3Aprint%2F+%2Durl%3Aindex%2F+%2Durl%3Aresources%2Fpronunciations+%2Durl%3Amultimedia%2F+%2Durl%3A%2Fprofessional%2Fau+%2Durl%3A%2Fprofessional%2Fag+%2Durl%3Alexicomp%2F&charset=utf8&la=en&start=0

Pain Management Guidelines (2009). *Pharmacological Management of Persistent Pain in Older Adults*. JAGS. 57(8).

Sangl, J. (2007). Pain Management in Nursing Homes-AHQR report. Retrieved December 26, 2010, from http://apha.confex.com/recording/apha/135am/pdf/free/4db77adf5df9fff0d3caf5cafe28f496/paper161190_0.pdf

WHO Ladder Guidelines (2010). Retrieved December 26, 2010, from http://www.painbalance.org/who-cancer-pain-relief-ladder-1297651989

Wikipedia (2010). Waddle sign. Retrieved December 16, 2010, from http://en.wikipedia.org/wiki/Waddell's_signs

Chapter 5
Eating Problems & Nutrition

Maintaining a healthy weight can be difficult for elders. A change in weight is often the first indicator of health problems in an elder. This chapter will discuss the changes elders experience with aging that affect weight, including changes in taste, the reduced caloric requirements many experience due to being less active, and problems resulting from health conditions that affect weight, such as loss of teeth, diabetes, heart failure, and kidney disease. Constipation is a major problem for many elders and can cause a great deal of discomfort. A discussion will follow of the causes of elimination problems (constipation and diarrhea) and ways to manage both pharmacologically, as well as through dietary and activity interventions.

Eating & Nutrition

Eating is essential for staying alive and being healthy. And eating, in our society, is more than just meeting nutritional needs – it is a form of socialization. It is something that is celebrated – people get together for holidays, birthdays, and special occasions. It is ritualistic – many have meals with 'the family' or with friends. And it is a source of enjoyment because most people like to eat different foods and go to different places according to food preferences.

Good health depends on eating right, especially in elders. Weight changes, particularly weight loss, can be an early indicator of health problems in an older person. Many older individuals are not as active as they were when younger, will require a smaller caloric intake and have some muscle loss, as well as weight loss. If an older person eats the same amount of food (takes in the same amount of calories) as when they were younger and less active (burning off fewer calories), the elder will increase their weight. But many older individuals decrease their intake due to requiring fewer calories because of a more sedentary lifestyle. Weight is generally fairly stable in most elders due to slower metabolism. An abrupt weight loss or progressive weight loss can be an indicator of worsening medical conditions. And on the other extreme, weight gain may indicate heart failure or kidney disease.

What Causes Changes in Eating for Elders?

Eating can be affected by changes in older adults, including aging changes that affect the ability to taste foods, dental issues such as caries or loss of teeth, diminished appetite, possible indigestion or nausea, and subtle changes in bowel functioning – both constipation and diarrhea. Eating is a complex process that requires an intact neurological system, physical abilities, and psychological intactness to remember the steps of eating, as well as to interpret the sensations of hunger and thirst. Eating is one of the last functions of the 'activities of daily living' to be lost by older individuals.

Common problems in elders that can cause weight loss

- Infection
- Anemia caused by iron deficiency, B12 deficiency, chronic disease, kidney disease and/or poor diet (also chronic use of certain medications can lead to anemia)
- Liver disease, Lung disease, and Heart disease
- Thyroid disease, Diabetes, and other endocrine disorders
- Malnutrition, Poor dietary intake
- Kidney disease (renal failure)
- Depression and Dementia with memory impairment
- Gastrointestinal disorders, including gastroesophageal reflux disorder (GERD) and irritable bowel syndrome (IBS)
- Cerebrovascular disease, including strokes
- Cancer (malignancy)

Indigestion is a common cause of a decrease in appetite for an elder. It is defined as discomfort in the upper abdomen, including bloating, belching and nausea. Symptoms might be felt occasionally or as often as daily.

Causes of Indigestion

- Types of foods: especially fatty or greasy foods, spicy foods
- Eating too quickly
- Too much caffeine, alcohol, chocolate, or too many carbonated beverages
- Smoking
- Nervousness and Emotional upset
- Medications, including antibiotics, aspirin and nonsteroidal anti-inflammatory drugs (NSAIDs)
- Other causes: ulcers, gallstones, infection, or possibly a more serious condition such as pancreatitis or cancer

NOTE: if the problem is chronic and does not subside with dietary & lifestyle management, seek evaluation from a healthcare practitioner.

Management of Indigestion

Lifestyle

- **Eat smaller, more frequent meals**. Large meals can cause more problems with indigestion. Encourage a person to chew food slowly and thoroughly.
- **No eating 3 hours before lying down.** Lying down allows stomach contents to back up into the esophagus and cause indigestion.
- **Avoid irritating foods which are triggers.** Decrease or avoid irritating foods such as fatty and spicy foods, carbonated beverages, chocolate, caffeine, and alcohol.
- **Smoking irritates the stomach and increases acid production**. Decrease or avoid smoking.
- **Maintain a healthy weight**. Excess weight puts pressure on a person's abdomen, pushing up the stomach and causing acid to back up into the esophagus.
- **Exercise regularly** to decrease weight, keep off extra weight, and promote better digestion.
- **Manage stress**. Create a calm environment at mealtime.

Medications to Manage Indigestion

- **Antacids** work by neutralizing stomach acid. Alka-Seltzer, Maalox, Mylanta, Rolaids, Riopan and others are available.
- **H-2-receptor antagonists (H2RAs)** reduce stomach acid and work

longer – but not as quickly – as antacids. These include nizatidine (Axid), cimetidine (Tagamet), famotidine (Pepcid) and ranitidine (Zantac), which are available over-the-counter or by prescription. Use cautiously since these medications can cause increased bruising or bleeding.

- **Proton pump inhibitors (PPIs)** reduce stomach acid and are stronger than H2RAs. Rabeprazole (Aciphex), esomeprazole (Nexium), lansoprazole (Prevacid), omeprazole (Prilosec), pantoprazole (Protonix), and omeprazole with sodium bicarbonate (Zegerid) are most effective for people who also have gastroesophageal reflux disease (GERD).
- **Antibiotics.** If the bacteria that causes peptic ulcer disease (Helicobacter pylori) is causing the problem, an antibiotic may be necessary.
- **Antidepressants.** If a thorough evaluation doesn't reveal a cause for the symptoms and the conventional treatments above don't work, a doctor may recommend an antidepressant medication.

Table 5-1. *Medications that can affect weight*	
Medication class	**Some of the possible side effects**
Anticholinergic drugs	Cognition changes – increases confusion, dysgeusia, dry mouth, anorexia, nausea
Antiepileptic drugs	Cognition changes – confusion, sedation, or agitation, anorexia, possibly overeating
Benzodiazepines	Anorexia, depression, cognition changes – confusion or sedation
Beta blockers	Cognition changes, depression
Central alpha antagonists	Cognition changes, anorexia, depression
Diuretics (high-potency combinations)	Dehydration, electrolyte abnormalities
Glucocorticoids	Steroid myopathy, diabetes, osteoporosis, agitation, anxiety, paranoia
More than four prescription medications	Drug interactions, adverse effects
Neuroleptics	Anorexia, parkinsonism
Opioids	Anorexia, cognition changes
SSRIs	Anorexia or weight gain
Tricyclic antidepressants	Dysgeusia, dry mouth, cognition changes

How do We Eat

Eating is a complex process and requires an intact cognitive status – an ability to interpret sensations of hunger and thirst, an ability to understand how to eat, and an ability to coordinate the steps of eating; an intact physical status – an ability to chew and swallow, intact and functioning cranial nerves, and functioning muscles to feed self; and an appetite.

Complexity of Eating (Steps of Eating)

Oral preparatory phase
- prepare the food into a bite small enough to place in the mouth so it can be chewed
- bring the food to the mouth

Oral phase – chew the food and prepare the bolus of food to swallow
- food is placed in the mouth and chewed
- food is mixed with saliva and reshaped by chewing it to a consistency that can be swallowed

Pharyngeal – swallowing
- breathing ceases momentarily as the bolus of food is moved through the pharynx
- the nasopharynx is sealed with the elevation of the soft palate
- the tongue pushes the bolus through the pharynx via sequential pressure waves
- just milliseconds before the onset of the pharyngeal contraction, the hyoid & larynx move upward to close the laryngeal vestibule and airway entrance, thereby preventing aspiration (saliva, food, or fluid entering the lungs)
- upper esophageal sphincter (UES) opens to allow the bolus to enter the esophagus
- as the bolus of food passes the UES, the pharyngeal structures return to rest and breathing begins again

Esophageal
- the food bolus moves to the stomach through muscular action – peristalsis which is the product of the reciprocal relaxation and contraction of the circular and longitudinal muscles that make up the esophagus
- Finally – at rest, the esophagus relaxes and is a collapsed, closed tube with a sphincter at each end

Aging Changes That Affect Eatting

Aging changes a person's body in many ways. In addition, factors such as an elder's decreasing ability to get around (which may decrease caloric requirements), potential arthritis (which can affect a person's ability to feed oneself), and sensory changes to taste and smell may combine with the cumulative negative impact on a person's ability to eat. Changes in the digestive tract also affect digestion and absorption of food; these changes include the acidity as well as the amount of gastric secretions and a slower motility of the intestines. Thus, some older individuals are at risk for malnutrition and unintended weight loss due to the physiological changes associated with normal aging (rd411, 2010).

How does Vision affect a Person's Ability to Eat?

There are many changes to a person's vision associated with normal aging that can affect eating, including a decreased ability to see objects that are close – a majority of older individuals develop farsightedness or presbyopia; for example, the person sees something in front of them but may be unaware of what the food is. Many older individuals have difficulty seeing objects of similar color; for example, light colored mashed potatoes disappear on a white plate. Also affected by aging is depth perception and this is more pronounced in individuals with Alzheimer's disease; for example, the person cannot estimate how much food is on their plate or may not realize that they have not eaten enough food. Untreated vision problems in older persons are also associated with an increased risk of decline in cognitive function and a hastening of the progression of certain dementias, including Alzheimer's disease (Bankhead, 2010).

Normal Aging Changes to Vision

- **Depth perception**: The cornea, which refracts light, becomes flatter, less smooth, and thicker – making older eyes more susceptible to astigmatism.
- **Decreased ability to differentiate colors**: There is a yellowing of the lens, which causes some reduction of the eye's ability to discriminate blues, greens, and violets; yellows, oranges, and reds are seen more clearly.

- **Ptosis:** Eyelids may droop as elasticity diminishes, leading to occlusion of the visual field.

- **Dry Eyes:** Decrease in orbicular muscle strength causes an eyelid to stay open slightly, leading to dryness of the eyes which, in turn, can lead to blurry vision.

- **Presbyopia:** After 40 years of life, the eye losses the ability to accommodate to see close objects as clearly and this problem continues to worsen or progress throughout a person's life. This makes it difficult for a person to identify the food on their plate.

- **Decreased Peripheral Vision:** Peripheral vision decreases, making a person's visual field smaller and causing difficulty in seeing approaching objects or people that are not directly in front of the person, or it can make items disappear (i.e., the person only sees the items in the center of the plate and foods on the edges may not be seen).

- **Slower Pupil Accommodation:** Pupil size is smaller, creating a slower constriction in the presence of bright light. There is a slowing of the pupil's dilation in dark settings and a slowing in the ability to accommodate to changes in light. Glare occurs often in sunlight, as well as in the reflections off shiny objects. Older eyes need three times more light, causing night vision to be impaired for older adults.

- **Glaucoma:** The anterior chamber of the eye decreases as the thickness of the lens increases. In some older individuals, there is an increase in the density of collagen fibers, which leads to inefficient resorption of intraocular fluids and glaucoma.

- **Cataracts:** Lens opacities can develop after the age of 50, causing a cloudiness in vision; this can progress to obscure vision completely and cause everything to appear blurred.

- **Opacities:** can develop and can be seen as spots or clusters of dots in the visual field. These are coalesced vitreous that have broken off the periphery or central part of the retina. They are largely harmless, although can be annoying and potentially cause visual hallucinations and paranoia.

NOTE: If an individual notices a sudden occurrence of spots and/or pain in the eye, this could be an indication of an emergent problem and requires immediate evaluation.

(Ebersole et al, 2004; Eye Digest, 2007; Tumosa, 2004)

How do Hearing and Auditory Distractions Affect Eating?

A noisy environment may make eating difficult for individuals who are easily distracted. Hearing deficits can add to this problem. Many individuals have some degree of hearing loss, making certain sounds and consonants difficult to hear – when trying to listen to conversations in their surroundings, they may only hear bits and pieces of words and conversations due to loss of the ability to hear certain sounds; this can lead to delusions and paranoia in some older individuals.

Auditory Distractions Affecting Eating
- Some individuals find it hard to keep the conversations in the same room
- Hearing deficits can cause fragmentation of conversations the person hears, making the person paranoid and suspicious
- Background noises cause distractions or frighten a person who does not understand what the sound is
  o ice machines
  o metallic clanging of silverware
  o announcements on the public-address system
  o a radio or boom box playing "dinner" music
  o Many individuals with dementia find it hard to cope with the stimulation associated with group dining

Changes to Taste & Smell in Normal Aging
A person's sense of taste and smell diminish with age. These two senses interact closely, helping an individual taste and appreciate food. People have approximately 8,000 taste buds, which have the primarily responsibity for sensing as well as differentiating sweet, salty, sour, and bitter tastes (Lembert, 2000). The number of taste buds decreases as individuals age, beginning at about age 40 to 50 in women and at 50 to 60 in men – the remaining taste buds also begin to atrophy or be lost. A person's ability to taste certain foods changes over time, making food preferences change.

The sense of smell enhances a person's ability to taste foods and, as the sense of smell diminishes with normal aging, the ability to taste foods will also change. The ability to smell begins at nerve receptors high in the membranes of the nose and, with normal wear and tear, these receptors can become dislodged and diminish a person's ability to smell. Although most older individual's have a decline in their sense of smell with normal aging, it has been found that this loss is more pronounced in individuals suffering from Alzheimer's disease. Smell (and to a lesser extent, taste) play a role in both safety and enjoyment. A delicious meal or pleasant aroma can improve social interaction and enjoyment of life. But certain smells can alert a person that something is not safe to eat or that something is not an edible object. NOTE: a sudden loss of smell could indicate a potential brain tumor and must be evaluated.

The ability to taste is typically lost in a standard pattern. Usually salty and sweet tastes are lost first, with bitter and sour tastes lasting slightly longer. Many older individuals will attempt to eat very salty foods and eat sweets frequently to satisfy their need for these tastes. Additionally, an older person's mouth produces less saliva with aging; this can cause a dry mouth, contributing to difficulty in swallowing. It also makes digestion slightly less efficient and can increase dental problems because, with an adequate amount of saliva, food particles are washed off teeth – without removal of food particles, there is an increased development of caries, which can lead to tooth breakage, tooth loss, gingivitis, and illness (MedLine Plus, 2010).

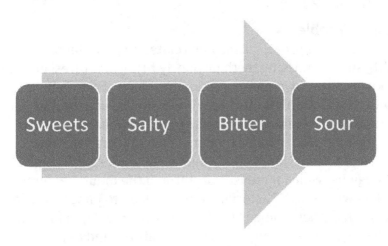

Figure 5-1. *Changes in Taste:*
Order in which an elder loses the ability to taste

Dysphagia

Dysphagia, chewing and/or swallowing problems, can be life threatening for certain older individuals. The muscles of the mouth and throat may no longer be working properly, allowing bits of food and liquid to be aspirated or inhaled into the lungs; this can lead to respiratory infections, pneumonia, and potentially death. Other factors contributing to dysphasia include a person's level of consciousness (how alert a person is), medications, distractions and certain eating patterns, such as taking abnormally large bites or not chewing adequately.

When a person aspirates either food or fluid, the passages of the lungs may become congested or blocked and the person may begin to choke. For frail, elderly individuals, a choking fit can be fatal. A person can also aspirate without showing apparent symptoms (like choking or coughing); this is referred to as 'silent aspiration'. Aspiration of food or fluid into the lungs can cause aspiration pneumonia, which is a potentially deadly problem. This can happen in individuals with dementia and is more prevalent in individuals who are in the final stage of the dementia process. Repeated bouts of aspiration pneumonia will weaken a person's system and may eventually lead to death (How to care, 2010).

Chewing Problems

Chewing problems may be related to poor dental health, such as missing teeth or poorly fitting dentures, muscle weakness or paralysis, or cognition problems. Factors that can lead to dental problems include diminished saliva production (which occurs commonly in elders). Certain medications can also dry a person's mouth. In many elders, dental caries or cavities can occur due to food stagnating on the teeth or poor oral hygiene, which increases bacteria in the mouth. Aspiration of saliva with a high bacterial count can lead to pneumonia in elders – and pneumonia is the leading cause of death for elders in nursing homes. Many elders have dentures and it must be realized that dentures do not fit the roof of the mouth until the dentures have been worn for an average of 9 to 12 months – the upper palate must form into the denture for the denture to fit snugly. It should also be noted that a change of 15% of person's weight will impact the proper fit of dentures – with weight loss, the denture may be too loose and it will fall or drop when the person opens their mouth to eat, which leads to inefficient chewing. Properly fitting dentures, proper oral hygiene before and after meals, and regular dental visits may help minimize some of these problems. Chewing problems may be obvious or may present with subtle symptoms, such as slower eating or diminished intake with meals.

Signs of chewing, swallowing, or potential aspiration problems

- Extra effort chewing or swallowing
- Eating very slowly
- Packing food into the cheeks
- Swallowing several times for a single mouthful of food
- Shortness of breath during eating
- Coughing or choking while eating or drinking
- Drooling
- Fluid or mucous leaking from the nose after swallowing
- A wet-sounding voice after eating
- Change in the quality of the voice after eating or drinking
- Increased congestion in the chest after eating
- Repeated bouts of pneumonia

If an individual is suspected of having problems with either overt aspiration (coughing or choking when drinking and/or eating) and/or has repeated bouts of respiratory infections and other signs of aspiration, attempt to identify what could be causing the problem:

- What was the person doing when the coughing/choking occurred – talking, laughing, or walking?
- What type of food or fluid was he/she eating when the coughing or choking occurred – thin liquids, breads, hard-to-chew meats?
- If the person wears dentures, were they being worn at the time of the choking episode? Do the dentures fit properly?

(How to Care, 2010)

Getting help

If there are concerns about a person's eating or drinking abilities, there are some key healthcare professionals who can offer advice and guidance:

- **Dietitians** – provide advice on issues such as poor appetite, weight loss or weight gain, food enrichment and vitamin and food supplements
- **Speech and language therapists** – give advice and guidance on swallowing difficulties.; it is important that changes to the texture of food are only made when necessary and with their professional advice
- **Occupational therapists** – advise on adapted eating aids, such as cutlery, cups and plate mats, that help to maintain independent eating

(rd411, Alzheimer's Association, 2010)

Assessing Eating Problems

When an individual is suspected of having problems eating or swallowing, an initial assessment is done to identify the nature of the problem, identify any contributing factors, differentiate physiologic impairment and/or cognitive factors, identify ways to improve safety, and identify the person's ability to benefit from skilled intervention. Assessment begins with identification of the problem and the effects it has on an older person. Initially, observation of a person's eating abilities will assist in obtaining a general understanding of the problem. The next step is an interview with the person to assist in identifying the problem. It is also helpful to obtain information from anyone who has observed the eating problem or episodes of trouble swallowing and/or dysphagia. During an individual interview with the person having eating difficulties, there are two key questions:

1. What are the problems with eating, drinking, and swallowing?
2. Why does the person think he/she is having a problem with swallowing?

The following information should be sought:
- all diagnoses, including any type of dementia with which the person has been diagnosed
- current weight, as well as any recent weight changes
  - weight assessment of the most recent 6 months to assess weight fluctuations or for a trend of continued weight loss
- diet and any recent changes
- eating habits, including food types and amounts consumed at scheduled & unscheduled times
- abilities to feed self throughout the course of each meal and throughout the day
- any eating and/or chewing difficulties
- signs/symptoms of hoarseness or wet-sounding voice after meals, runny nose after meals, congestion, coughing, choking with drinking or taking medications, fever, and lethargy
- if available – any radiological test results (chest and modified barium swallow)
- history of respiratory infections and/or pneumonia

An assessment of the person's functional status and cognitive abilities is imperative. This assessment should include establishing abilities of recent recall and the ability to follow instructions, although this may be limited in individuals with memory impairment, dementia, or other language deficits. Elders with memory impairment may forget how to eat, forget the steps of eating, or may not be able to recognize food as food. After an assessment of a person's abilities, it is necessary to examine many other factors including: sensory function, head and neck positioning, oral motor skills, and swallowing skills like patterns of mastication (chewing), salivation, and laryngeal elevation (Curfman, 2005).

Treatment strategies will be influenced by many factors: information about a person's perception of the problem, cognitive status, and ability to understand and follow directions, and ability to learn new information. Many individuals with dementia who have dysphagia may have a neurologic impairment that will make the person unable to understand questions or unable to follow instructions. This may hinder participation in the assessment phase and hinder their ability to learn how to prevent the problem. Expressive aphasia is an inability to verbalize what a person is thinking and Receptive aphasia is an inability to understand what they are being told. Sensory function: It is important to determine whether a person has problems with sensory pathways. Some sensory problems that may contribute to a decrease in a person's intake can be an altered or absent perception of taste, an inability to sense hot food (leading to potential/actual injuries of the mouth), and/or profound sensory loss in the later stages of the dementia that hinders a person's ability to chew and swallow.

The following six anatomic sites are assessed to determine if a sensory deficit is causing problems with eating:
- tongue (anterior two-thirds)
- tongue (posterior one-third)
- hard palate
- soft palate
- posterior pharyngeal wall
- laryngeal region

(Curfman, 2005)

Head and neck positioning: Body position while eating is an important factor to assess – both the body position (sitting or lying) as well as the position of the person's head (flexed at a 90 degree position or head back while in a lying position). A person may require assistance in positioning and caregivers should be assessed in how they position an individual for mealtimes. Three common head/neck positions that occur in certain advanced illnesses as well as the later stages of dementia include:

1. chronic head/neck flexion (head bent forward)
2. variable head/neck flexion/extension caused by a lack of positioningmanagement (inability to hold head upright)
3. chronic head/neck hyperextension (head positioned backward)

Oral motor skills: Visual assessment of an individual's eating ability consists of watching and assessing motion and movement, strength, and coordination of oral structures (lips, tongue – anterior, middle, and posterior, and soft palate). Additional assessment of the functional movement patterns required for the oral stage of swallowing include assessing manipulation of food during chewing, cohesive food bolus formation, anterior-to-posterior transit of cohesive food bolus, and later stage of swallowing – the transfer or moving of the food bolus into the pharynx.

Pattern of Chewing (mastication): Assessment of mastication involves assessing the muscles associated with chewing and the pattern of chewing as well as swallowing. If an individual has facial weakness or paralysis, the pattern of chewing may be altered. The function of the oral musculature will determine the pattern of chewing, which will deteriorate in a predictable fashion with the progression of the disease if an individual has dementia. The progressive deterioration in the mastication patterns shown below reflex integration to lower level reflex integration during the detrioration of the ability to chew, more pronounced in individuals with dementia:

• rotary chew pattern
• lateral chew/chomping pattern and jaw-jerk reflex
• suck-swallow pattern
• absent oral motor function for chewing

(Curfman, 2005)

Salivation: Salivation is important to add moisture to food in order to make it more easily swallowed. Assessment of salivary function includes inspecting the oral mucosa visually to determine adequacy of saliva flow, review of medications that can cause decreased saliva production, and review of medical history for conditions that can affect saliva production. There are many common medications that can reduce salivation, including medications such as anticholinergic agents, antidepressants, and antipsychotic drugs. If salivary flow is adequate, the mouth will appear moist; if hyposalivation (low salivary production) occurs, the oral cavity will become dry. Symptoms of dry mouth, also known as xerostomia include mouth pain, difficulty chewing, difficulty swallowing, weight loss, mouth infections, tooth decay, a dry, cracked tongue, bleeding gums, cracked corners of the mouth, badly fitting dentures, and dryness in the eyes, nose, skin, and throat. If a person appears to have a dry mouth or complains about a dry mouth, the person should be assessed for signs of dehydration, including dry mucous membranes, loss of skin turgor, intense thirst, flushed skin, oliguria (decreased urine output), concentrated urine (which appears as dark yellow or brown in color), and/or possible elevated temperature (Curfman, 2005).

Analyzing volitional swallows and laryngeal elevation: Once swallowing is initiated, it should occur rapidly. The person observing should assess if elevation of the larynx occurs during swallowing. Assessment encompassing observation of the components of laryngeal elevation would include the speed of laryngeal elevation, the movement of the structures involved, and the integrity of their movement.

Cognitive Impairment or Dementia effects on eating in elders
Memory Issues can affect an elder's ability to eat: There are many reasons why older individuals who may be experiencing memory impairment decrease their intake. Loss of memory and problems with judgment can cause decreased food intake:

- Problems with shopping – inability to decide what to buy or unable to make appropriate food selections
- Inability to cook – unable to understand how the stove works, how to prepare food, carry out a recipe, or how to recognize utensils
- Inability to eat – sometimes the damage to the brain may affect the person's ability to carry out the sequential steps of eating

An individual suffering from dementia may have declining mental as well as physical abilities which will have an effect on nutrition and hydration throughout the course of the person's illness. In the early stage of dementia, an individual may forget to eat, may become depressed and not want to eat, or may become distracted and leave the table without eating. As the disease progresses, the individual with dementia may be easily distracted and unable to sit long enough to eat. Yet at this stage, a person may require an additional 600 calories per day because of wandering and motor restlessness, while other individuals may be less active, possibly chair bound or bed bound and require fewer calories. In the late stage of a dementia, an individual may forget the sequence of steps to eating and may not have intact oral motor skills for chewing and swallowing, leading to malnourishment and the initiation of a cascade of decline. This can cause a person to begin to 'waste away' (Curfman, 2005).

In many individuals suffering from dementia, there can be problems with the appetite center. Some of the different problems include: a) Overeating or insatiable appetite – consider offering 5 or 6 small meals per day; have low-calorie snacks available; distract the person with other activities such as walking or singing; and it may be necessary to lock up some foods; b) Under-eating – consider offering a glass of juice or wine to stimulate appetite; offer ice-cream or egg nogs; increase exercise; try offering all or more of one food before offering the next to avoid change of taste and texture; have the largest meal coincide with the time of the day when the person is at their best – usually the middle of the day; offer familiar or favorite foods; and c) Sweet cravings – consider offering milk shakes or egg nogs as an alternative; offer low calorie ice-cream and high protein 'sweets', or sweets made with whole grains and vegetables (myDoc, 2010).

In some individuals, hunger sensations may no longer be interpreted by the damaged brain and a person is unaware of the necessity to eat. The person may forget they have already eaten and are always seeking food or forget to eat at all. And some medications, as well as concurrent medical problems a person can have, may cause potential side effects that affect appetite or cause nausea and/or indigestion.

Dysphagia of Dementia

The following are secondary conditions related to the primary diagnosis of dementia:

- absent oral motor pattern for chewing
- poor sensory awareness
- negative reaction to food textures and consistencies
- suck-swallow mastication pattern
- significant irreversible pharyngeal dysphagia
- reduced intake by mouth secondary to behavioral issues

Treatment in Individuals with Dementia and Dysphagia

There are ways to improve dysphagia in individuals with dementia. Treatment can be divided into direct treatment, preferably by a trained professional – usually a speech therapist who works directly with a person, teaching strategies to improve the problem: sensory stimulation, diet modification, muscle strengthening, and caregiver training in feeding assistance. And indirect treatment is an individualized plan of care which incorporates environmental modifications, adaptive equipment/assistive devices, and safety strategies to be used by a designated caregiver: addition of sweetener to food items (if the person prefers sweet tastes); use of alternative nutritional systems, such as enteral feeding (feeding a person through a tube inserted directly into the stomach); and/or oral care/sensory stimulation provided by caregiver (Curfman, 2005).

Treatment suggestions in Individuals with Dementia/Dysphagia:

- sensory stimulation
  - o increase texture variation (dry crackers or crisp cookies)
  - o increase mouth sensation
  - o facilitate mastication (chewing) pattern
- diet management (as prescribed), development of an individualized plan of care/functional maintenance program, and caregiver training to maximize an individual's abilities to maintain the highest level of function
- provide oral care before meals with a citric swab to increase salivation
- offer small frequent meals throughout the day
- offer high-calorie, high protein finger foods throughout the day to increase

intake of calories
- offer water frequently throughout the day to increase hydration
- evaluate for appropriate positioning to expedite safe, effective swallow function & meal completion
- provide mouth care after every meal

(Curfman, 2005)

Distraction

Many older adults are easily distracted when eating, which can lead to malnutrition and other problems such as aspiration. Imagine being in a busy restaurant with a group of friends, there is loud music playing close or the elder is sitting in a busy area with people walking by frequently. There is a lot of activity and the conversations around the table are loud. Ordering requires making a choice from a long list of options on the menu as well as keeping up with the conversations at the table. The waiter is hovering and a person feels pressure to order. It may be a challenging to concentrate on the conversations around the table while choosing from the menu, but will manage to make a decision, order, and continue to converse with the people at the table despite everything else going on.

For many elders, especially those individuals with dementia, a noisy environment can be confusing: it can further increase difficulty in a person's ability to concentrate and focus. Some individuals with dementia cannot tolerate this type of environment and feel compelled to escape – some are able to do this and maneuver away. But others cannot and are trapped, possibly becoming overwhelmed by their surroundings. Being aware that individuals with dementia are overwhelmed when over-stimulated by their environment and understanding that these individuals may struggle to concentrate at mealtimes if there are distractions, will assist caregivers in developing an appropriate meal-time environment for these individuals. It is encouraged that a confused person's eating environment be calm and relaxed with minimal distractions, if possible (SCIE, 2010).

Eating Environment can hinder eating for individuals with dementia:

- Activity
- Noise
- Distractions (conversations, shows, music, people walking by)
- Lighting
- Seating (friendship, need for assistance to eat, etc)
- Choices of foods
- Differing diets at the same table

Individuals suffering from dementia may not feel relaxed and comfortable eating with other people or in an unfamiliar environment. Others may have difficulty eating food due to frequent spills or just become paranoid. Any of these issues can only make feelings of embarrassment worse if sitting with others. As a result, the person may leave food uneaten even when hungry. Allow a person to sit and eat in a place where they feel comfortable, either at a table or perhaps sitting with a tray on their lap in a comfortable chair. Remember socialization is encouraged to keep a person interacting with others as well as for safety reasons – to prevent a person from choking and no-one being aware of the problem if the person was eating alone (SCIE, 2010).

Encouraging Eating in the Early & Mid Stages of Dementia

In the early to middle stages of an elder's dementia, including Alzheimer's dementia, many things can occur that may cause an eating problem for the individual. The ability to taste foods changes normally as an individual ages and this is more pronounced in individuals with Alzheimer's disease and certain other dementias, which can lead to cravings for sweets. Mealtimes can present many challenges. A person with dementia may have changes in appetite, loss of interest in food, may forget to eat or that he or she has already eaten. But on a more basic level, the individual may have trouble differentiating what is food and what isn't, as well as problems in knowing what to do with utensils and even what to do with the food.

Table 5-2. *Eating Problems in Elders with Different Dementias*		
Alzheimer's Disease	**Parkinson's Disease Dementia**	**Frontotemporal Dementia**
Anosmia • diminished sense of smell Ability to taste of food diminished •Prefers highly seasoned, spicy, & sweet foods because they are more satisfying Food preferences change Need to change consistency of food to enhance swallowing abilities Easily distracted •May need prompting	50-60% of individuals with Parkinson's disease experience problems with eating at some point Oral Lingual tremor at rest Multiple lingual gestures during oral bolus manipulation & propulsion Pharyngeal Decreased laryngeal elevation Incomplete upper esophageal sphincter relaxation Pharyngeal residual after swallowing Decreased muscle tone	Increased appetite with increased sweet cravings Abnormal oral behaviors •Atypical bite sizes •Decreased chewing •Eating non-edible things Involuntary bolus movement to the pharynx or into the unclosed airway before the elicitation of a swallow

Managing Early Eating Problems in Elders

Here are some ways to assist the person to eat a nutritious meal:

1. **Difficulty in Recognition:** Mark plates and utensils so it is clear that they belong to the individual since some individuals may have great difficulty in knowing which plate is theirs. Have the person sit in the same place for each meal so they can develop a sense of familiarity.

2. **Locate a comfortable place to eat:** Some individuals are not comfortable eating at a dining table – try to allow the person to eat where they most comfortable with the plate and utensils as long as the person has someone near to prevent aspiration. Have the table at a good height for the person and have everything within reaching distance for the person. Attempt to have the person sitting upright in as close to the usual posture of sitting in a chair for eating at a table.

3. **Do not allow the person to eat alone:** An elder should not eat alone, some may forget to eat and need prompting (or reminding to eat); some put food in their mouths and forget the food is there (a potential choking hazard); and some do not realize the need to eat and just need reminding. Eating is a form of socialization and eating with others helps a person stay connected with their community.

4. **Distractions can hinder eating:** Serve meals in a quiet place so that an elder can focus on eating. Turn off distractions such as the television, radio, or overhead paging system. Keep the table setting simple – remove flowers, centerpieces and condiments. Use only the utensils needed for the meal.

5. **Encourage healthy snacking:** Many elders, especially those with dementia, develop an affinity for sweets. Caregivers may try to steer away from sweets because of concerns about proper nutrition but this can be used as an advantage: bake cookies with high protein additives, oatmeal, dried fruits and veggies; oatmeal cookies have excellent fiber and oatmeal can be added to anything to aid in nutrition; pumpkin and squash can be used to make a bar cookie; and there are many high protein snacks that are sweet tasting.

6. **Make foods palliative:** Monitor smells in the environment if a person seems to get nauseated with certain odors. Check the food temperature because a person may eat better if the food is served at its appropriate temperature. Some individuals also have difficulty in telling if a food or beverage is too hot to eat or drink.

7. **Overwhelmed by choices:** In individuals who are overwhelmed by choices and may be unable to choose when offered too many selections – serve only one or two foods at a time. Consider serving one food at a time such as mashed potatoes followed by chicken tenders.

8. **Enhance foods with spices:** Due to the changes in an elder's taste buds, food preferences will change. The ability to taste salt usually is lost early and it may not be appropriate to add more salt to an older person's diet (unless contraindicated due to other disease processes) – food may taste better when it is spiced up (which makes it more flavorful).

9. **Control intake of snacks:** Place snack foods and finger foods in one area of the kitchen, so that they are easy to find and make sure that available foods are nutritious. Apples, carrots, and celery sticks make excellent foods to leave out where individuals may help themselves to the nutritious snacks – be cautious if an elder chokes easily or is prone to not chewing food adequately.

10. **Helping differentiate between food and non-foods:** A decline in vision can make foods unrecognizable for some elders and some foods may not be visualized as readily if the food is similar in color to the plate. Some elders with dementia will find it difficult to tell what is edible and what isn't, which can result in them eating napkins, artificial or plastic fruits, bar soap, cleaning supplies, or just about anything that can be placed in a person's mouth. This can be potentially very dangerous. Use the same caution with all dangerous materials and consider child-locks on cabinets to prevent ingestion of hazardous materials.

11. **Assist with handling of plates and utensils:** Elders with arthritis, tremors, or movement disorders, as well as those with a diagnosis of dementia, will have progression in the disease and the individual may have difficulty in using knives, forks, spoons and cups – the person may spill food, drop food or drinks, or have problems coordinating the use of utensils. As a person loses the ability to manipulate silverware, provide finger foods as much as possible. Some foods, however, do not lend themselves to being eaten with fingers, so help by spooning it into a person's mouth may be needed. Put the person's hand on your hand with the spoon as you fed him/her. Cups can be a big problem due to spills or because the person may forget from which end to drunk – consider using some kid cups with a heavy duty built-in straw or a sippy cup with large handles.

12. **Dealing with hidden foods:** Foods can sometimes disappear for an elder with either visual impairment or dementia – the foods may seem to disappear or run together. Consider using heavy plastic plates that have divided compartments and high sides or a lip on the edge, so the food is visible and it is not accidentally shoved off the plate (and

disappears for the person). Some individuals will also hide food with their personal effects. Leaving snacks out can become a problem, yet snack foods may still be in demand. But limiting the amount of snack foods left out is better. Observe where the person's favorite hiding spots are located and check them when food seems to disappear. Then it is simple to remove food and other inappropriate items the person may have hidden.

13. **Encourage adequate fluid intake:** Don't overlook the importance of fluids. Water is essential to prevent dehydration and urinary tract infections. Adding liquid meal replacements and supplements such as Ensure or an Instant Breakfast to a person's meal is a wonderful way of adding calories as well as fluids, vitamins, and nutrients. (Water in tea or coffee is not a good substitute for plain water because these drinks have caffeine, which can act as a diuretic and cause the person to urinate and worsen dehydration.) Remember to encourage the person to drink plenty of water throughout the day.

14. **Choking hazards:** Avoid nuts, popcorn, hard candy, and gum. These foods can get caught in one's throat. Be alert for symptoms of choking and learn how to perform the Heimlich maneuver, just in case the person has choking problems. (Alzheimer's Association, 2010; Knox, 2010)

Encourage Independence for Individuals with Dementia (Do Not Encourage Dependence)

- Make the most of the person's abilities. Allow a person to eat from a bowl instead of a plate or use a plate with a lip around the edge, or allow a person to eat with a spoon instead of a fork – even with their hands, if it's easier.

- Serve finger foods. Chicken fingers, potato wedges, cheese cubes, cherry tomatoes, etc. are easier to pick up with one's hands and manipulate or to eat on the go.

- Demonstrate how to eat or use a "watch me" technique. Offer a demonstration of how to eat: hold a spoon, and make the motion of eating or eat with the person and show the person how to eat by example.

- Don't worry about neatness. Let individuals feed themselves as much as possible. Consider getting plates with suction cups and no-spill glasses.

Table Strategies For Managing Eating Problems with Dementia and Dysphagia

FORGETFULNESS AND DISORIENTATION

UNABLE TO IDENTIFY THE SENSATION OF HUNGER AND THE NEED FOR FOOD

- Offer liquids and water consistently throughout the day – Dehydration may trigger increased combativeness and urinary tract infections, which can further the problems with eating
- Place beverage bars in places frequented by the person to encourage a person to drink more often

PLAYS WITH FOOD/FORGETS HOW TO EAT/DOES NOT RECOGNIZE FOOD – does not transition from the before-meal activity to the meal itself, thus continues to play with food because the person does not realize it is time to eat

- Offer environmental interventions to signal the change to eating, including altering the appearance of the table, such as a tablecloth, flowers, baskets for napkins, and place mats

EATS WITH FINGERS INSTEAD OF UTENSILS

- Increase the number of finger foods being offered
- Serve hot cereal or soups in a mug, or cut fresh fruits and vegetables into bite-size pieces
- Offer portable items such as breakfast bars, finger gelatin, and 'edible containers' such as ice cream cones as options
- Continue to try to encourage eating with utensils if the individual's skill level can be advanced

DOES NOT USE UTENSILS CORRECTLY – Limit the number of utensils – Often individuals with dementia eat with a knife because it is picked up with the dominant hand to cut food [whether needed or not] and then the person forgets to put it down to select a fork or spoon. Have food prepared and cut into bite size portions, then place a spoon or fork for the person to use.

TOO MANY CHOICES – A person is unable to make choices if too much food or too many containers are present at one time

- Serve one course at a time so that the necessity of making choices is limited and there are fewer distractions
- When appropriate, allow menu selection and the choice between two or three main courses

- If dining at a restaurant, offer the menu and give the cueing needed to help with choices. For example, 'Would you prefer chicken or the meatloaf today?' If individuals cannot make choices at all and you know their food preferences, make suggestions, 'They have great chicken and dumplings here. Would you like to try the chicken and dumplings for lunch?'

OVERWHELMED BY TOO MUCH FOOD – If the person feels that there is too much food on their plate, use two plates, serving half a meal at a time

DEMONSTRATES AN INABILITY TO UNDERSTAND WHAT IS EXPECTED AT MEALTIME – Establish the same routine at each meal
- Reinforce with simple one-step directions using visual and gestural cueing
- Placement of the fork/spoon in the resident's preferred hand
- Hand-over-hand caregiver assistance may trigger the eating process

LIMITED ATTENTION SPAN – Has an inability to stay focused on the task of eating, limiting the meal from being consumed entirely
- Use simple, concrete words
- Touch and redirect the person to continue eating
- Offering five or six meals per day may be needed for individuals who are unable to eat much at any one time, if they become agitated when caregivers attempt to refocus them

LEAVES THE TABLE DURING THE MEAL – The meal may be a combination of sitting and eating, followed by walking and eating finger foods from a bowl
- Make sandwiches with anything that will hold together
- Waist pouches may help someone who paces, to keep their hands free so they can hold finger foods

JUDGMENT AND SAFETY

EATS FOOD PIECES THAT ARE TOO BIG TO SWALLOW SAFELY
- Assess food pieces for size, thickness, and consistency and make necessary adjustments
- Consider providing precut meats and other food items cut into bite-size pieces

EATS NONEDIBLES
- Avoid garnishes that are not easily chewed or eaten and those that are decorative in nature

POURS LIQUIDS ONTO FOODS
- Offer only food and when finished, offer water and fluids

TAKES ANOTHER PERSON'S FOOD
- Offer visual cueing for boundaries by using place mats to reduce interest in another's meal
- Square tables provide better definition of territory than round tables

MANAGING PERCEPTUAL PROBLEMS IN ELDERS

VISION – Has difficulty discriminating boundaries between items
- Focus on color contrast in terms of the food to the plate or cup, and the contrast of the plate to the place mat (Supporting visual interpretation can reduce an elder's anxiety)
- Increase lighting in order so the person can see the food more clearly, since an older person's eyes need more lighting than a younger person's eyes
- Monitor for glare – may need to use indirect light
- If a person has had a stroke or is visually impaired on one side, consider placing a person's plate more to the person's good side so they can see the food more clearly

COMMUNICATION – Understanding and being understood
- Develop a list of food preferences and dislikes
- Use sensory cueing with frequent gestures and pointing
- Remove a food or an item away from the table and then bring it back, or remove the food from the plate to regain attention
- Use verbal encouragement, such as, 'This really tastes good, would you please try it and tell me what you think?'
- When asking questions about food choices, use 'either/or' questions rather than 'yes/no' questions which could lead to "no's" and not eating

WEIGHT GAIN/LOSS
- Providing large meals or double servings at the meals the person eats the best (such as breakfast) may help to maintain weight
- Offer small frequent meals or snacks between meals and before bedtime
- Alternate hot and cold foods to help trigger swallowing
- Enhance food tastes – consider using honey and sugar to enhance the taste of foods, if medically appropriate; sweet taste receptors remain intact through the end stage; therefore, residents with end-stage disease usually favor sweets and can be enticed to eat by adding sweet thickeners to foods
- Offer high-protein and high calorie foods

ANXIETY

- Sometimes elders become obsessed about seating placement – they may say someone is seated 'in my place' or demand the same seat every time and will become aggressive if someone else sits 'in my seat' – Consider using name cards, or remove the individual's seat until just before the person arrives at the table
- Sits too close to others or someone he/she dislikes – Be aware of a person's preferred tablemates, since an acceptable peer group is important to many individuals

CONCERNS AND PRIDE

- Delusions – Sometimes individuals with dementia have false beliefs: The person believes they have no money to pay for a meal: consider issuing meal tickets or 'credit cards'; have a bill filled out with a receipt – that helps an individual with 'no money' to accept the meal and pay later
- Offer color play money for elders to use, or tell them the meal is paid for by insurance
- Inform them that the meal is part of the 'club' membership; therefore, it is required that the person eat dinner at the club

DINING AREA – environment & equipment

- Some individuals may behave disruptively because of room size and setup, type and size of tables, lighting, window glare, dishes, glassware, or utensils
- Have a variety of tables available to meet specific, individualized needs
- A table for one or two may be needed if an individual with dementia is experiencing hostility or paranoia
- Square tables create a sense of 'my space'; round tables create the illusion of someone eating off another's plate
- Glare from windows or lights can create agitation; if feasible, provide natural sunlight
- Provide cups and glassware that are easy to grasp
- Consider serving soups and hot cereals in a mug or soup bowl with handles
- Use special cups with large handles and built-in straws for individuals who spill a lot

(Alzheimer's Association, 2010)

Enteral Feeding and End-of-Life Decisions

Some elders may consider a feeding tube to allow food, fluids, and medications to be provided. In those elders with physiological diseases that cause an inability to swallow, such as strokes, neuromuscular disorders, or advanced Parkinson's disease – a feeding tube may be necessary. Individuals with paralysis of the throat, or those who have had a stroke, may require a feeding tube to allow adequate hydration and nutrition while preventing aspiration of food and fluids. Some individuals with a diagnosis of dementia will advance to the terminal stages and will decrease their intake of food and water. Use of feeding tubes in the advanced stages of dementia is controversial and caregivers should be educated on the realistic expectations of inserting a feeding tube. Many elders with dementia have a feeding tube placed with inappropriate expectations of the outcomes.

Discussions surrounding feeding tubes being used to sustain life in the final stage of any disease, including dementia, should include the individual and family early in the person's disease, if possible, to determine what a person would wish to be done. It is better to have the person's input while the person is able to state his/her own preference regarding feeding tube use before he/she has lost the ability to communicate. If an elder can no longer participate in these discussions, it is important to provide caregivers with adequate information regarding available treatment options, what a feeding tube can and cannot do, and the consequences related to inserting a feeding tube or choosing not to place one, as well as alternatives for nutritional intake (Curfman, 2005).

Insertion of a feeding tube

A feeding tube inserted through the abdominal wall into the stomach is known as a percutaneous gastrostomy tube or percutaneous endoscopic gastrostomy tube (PEG tube); a tube inserted into the small intestine is known as a jejunostomy tube (J tube). Feeding tubes are used on a long-term basis; fluids, liquid nutrition, and medications can be given to a person through these tubes. Insertion of a PEG tube usually takes less than an hour and is done while the person is sedated. A small opening is made through the skin and the tube is inserted into the stomach. A PEG tube is inserted through this opening and secured in place.

Risks of the procedure

Putting in a feeding tube is usually a simple procedure. There are several potential problems which could occur, including bleeding, infection, skin irritation or leakage around the tube, nausea and vomiting, and diarrhea due to use of liquid feedings. Problems occur in less than 10% of individuals in the first few weeks after the procedure. Long range problems can include diarrhea, aspiration of the stomach contents, and/or problems with the tube (i.e., the tube getting blocked or being pulled out or falling out).

What can a feeding tube do?

It is important to define the overall goals of care and what a feeding tube can and cannot do. Some of the goals of using a feeding tube include improving a person's nutritional status, preventing aspiration, being able to give medications, and keeping a person comfortable. Feeding tubes are often placed in individuals who have had a stroke, Parkinson's disease, or other problems which affect swallowing. However, individuals with advanced dementia generally do not gain a significant amount of weight or have improved physical function when a feeding tube is placed. Feeding tubes also do not help wounds heal to a significant degree or prevent the occurrence of new pressure sores in frail elders who are incontinent (Ersek & Hanson, 2009). Aspiration pneumonia is a common complication of a well-hydrated individual or in a person with a feeding tube who has excessive contents in their stomach; aspiration may occur if the person vomits or has some of the contents reflux up the esophagus and into the lungs. This aspiration can lead to pneumonia and death in frail individuals with advanced dementia. And while prevention of aspiration is a goal of tube feeding, studies have shown that individuals with advanced dementia who have feeding tubes placed still continue to aspirate at the same rate as before the tube was placed.

Individuals who have a feeding tube placed are more likely to be hospitalized and have to go through painful procedures. Finally, a person who has a feeding tube must sometimes have their extremities forcefully restrained to keep the person from pulling out their feeding tube.

Will a feeding tube prolong life in advanced dementia?

The decision to use a feeding tube or not use a feeding tube can be difficult. The answer to the question should be based on personal preference, guided by available scientific evidence. Research indicates that there is no conclusive evidence on the benefits of feeding tubes in individuals with advanced dementia. Several studies have compared dementia patients with and without feeding tubes and most studies have found that a feeding tube does not prolong life for individuals with advanced dementia. Most individuals with feeding tubes do not survive very long; there are several studies that show that 20-30% of individuals who get feeding tubes die within a month after placement and 50-60% die within a year (Ersek & Hanson, 2009). Feedings tubes do extend life in individuals who have a mechanical problem with swallowing, due to such causes as strokes, advanced Parkinson's disease, or neurodegenerative disorders that result in severe muscle weakness affecting one's swallowing.

Other options beyond feeding tube placement for a person with dementia

If a person has decreased intake or has a decreased appetite caused by infection, constipation, or depression, then these conditions should be treated to see if the person's appetite improves. If a loss of appetite is caused by a side effect of a medication, then the medicine causing the problem may require a change, if possible. If a person can still chew and swallow, caregivers may wish to continue to assist the person with eating and, if necessary, hand feed the person. Often, the diet is modified and a person is given foods that are easy to eat. One important benefit of hand feeding is that it is a time for caregivers and families to interact with a person with dementia.

At this time, the person should be fed favorite foods, so that eating is a pleasant experience for the person.

In the late stage of dementia, an elder may be unable to sit upright, unable to swallow effectively, unable to understand instructions, and unable to remember how to chew and swallow. The main goal of care in the late stage of dementia is to improve an individual's ability to eat through the use of adaptive equipment or assistive devices. Caregivers are encouraged to attempt to maintain an individual in an upright position while eating: sitting upright with the head flexed at a 90 degree angle to simulate as closely as possible the way a person has eaten most of their lives.

Even when people with late-stage dementia can no longer eat because of swallowing problems, the person may be able to take small tastes of their favorite foods and beverages. Appropriate mouth care is important to maintain the person's oral hygiene and comfort. Other care includes treating pain and other symptoms, and providing emotional and spiritual support for the person and family. Many people with advanced dementia who cannot eat and drink qualify for hospice care, which can be provided in a home setting or a nursing home (Ersek & Hanson, 2009).

Chapter 5 References

Alzheimer's Association. (2010). Eating. Retrieved April 12, 2010, from http://www.alz.org/living_with_alzheimers_eating.asp

Bankhead, C. (2010). Old-Age vision problems linked to Dementia. MedPage Today. Retrieved April 17, 2010, from http://www. medpagetoday.com/Geriatrics/GeneralGeriatrics/18633

Curfman, S. (2005). Managing dysphagia in residents with dementia: skilled intervention for a common—and troubling—disorder. Nursing Homes. Retrieved 4-13-2010, from http://findarticles.com/p/articles/ mi_m3830/is_8_54/ai_n15338409/

Curfman, S. (2010). Managing Dysphagia in Residents with Dementia: SKILLED INTERVENTION FOR A COMMON—AND TROUBLING— DISORDER. Nursing Homes/Long Term Care Management. Retrieved April 12, 2010, from http://www.wrightstuff.biz/madyinrewide.html

Ersek, M., & Hanson, L. (2009). Tube Feeding Decisions for People with Advanced Dementia. AGS Foundation. Retrieved April 17, 2010, from http://www.healthinaging.org/public_education/pef/tube_feeding.php

How to Care. (2010). Eating and Nutrition. Retrieved April 18, 2010, from http://www.howtocare.com/diet2.htm

Knox, E. (2010). Tips on...Eating (Early and Middle Stages of Dementia). Retrieved April 12, 2010, from http://www.ec-online.net/knowledge/ Articles/eatingtip1.html

MedLine Plus. (2010). Aging Changes to the Senses. Retrieved April 17, 2010, from http://www.nlm.nih.gov/medlineplus/ency/ article/004013.htm

myDoc. (2010). Dementia and eating difficulties. Retrieved April 12, 2010, from http://www.mydr.com.au/seniors-health/dementia-and-eating-difficulties

rd411 (2010) Effects of eating habits and nutrition. Retrieved December 17, 2010, from http://rd411.com/index.php?option=com_conte nt&view=article&id=252:effects-of-aging-on-eating-habits-and-nutrition&catid=113:clinical-inservices&Itemid=381

SCIE. (2010) Eating well for people with dementia. Retrieved April 17, 2010, from http://www.scie.org.uk/publications/dementia/eating/ environment.asp

Chapter 6

Elimination
(Constipation and Other Issues)

Constipation is a major problem for many elders and can cause a great deal of discomfort. This chapter will present a discussion of the causes of elimination problems (constipation as well as diarrhea) and ways to manage both pharmacologically, as well as with dietary and activity changes..

~

Bowel habits vary considerably from one individual to another and are affected by age, physiology, diet, and social and cultural influences. Normal stool frequency ranges from 2 to 3 each day to 2 to 3 each week. The key to determining if there is an issue is a change in bowel elimination patterns – changes in stool frequency, consistency, volume, or composition (i.e., presence of blood, mucus, pus, or excess fatty material) which may indicate disease (Merck Manual, 2010).

Common abdominal problems in elders and what to do

Indigestion is discomfort in the upper abdomen including bloating, belching and nausea. Symptoms might be felt occasionally or as often as daily – see the previous chapter for a discussion on indigestion.

Bloating, burping and passing gas are natural and are usually caused by swallowed air or the breakdown of food through digestion. The problem may only happen occasionally or it may occur repeatedly in a single day. When gas and gas pains interfere with a person's daily activities, it may be an indication of something serious. To reduce bloating, it may help to avoid or reduce the intake of gas-producing foods. Many foods cause gas, including baked beans, broccoli, Brussels sprouts, cabbage, carbonated drinks, cauliflower, chewing gum, hard candy and fruits (such as apples, peaches and pears); limit or avoid these items if they appear to be the cause of frequent bloating and discomfort.

Abdominal pain is pain and discomfort that occurs in the abdomen – the areas of the torso between the chest and the pelvis. Everyone experiences abdominal pain periodically. Abdominal pain can be mild or severe, and it may be continuous or intermittent. Abdominal pain has many potential causes that aren't serious, such as gas pains or a pulled muscle. Anyone who presents with abdominal pain that is severe or that occurs over a long period of time should have the problem investigated by a healthcare practitioner.
(MayoClinic, 2010)

CONSTIPATION

Constipation is a common symptom affecting nearly 20% of the aging population (ACG, 2005). The prevalence by elders making an office visit to a healthcare provider for this problem outnumbers complaints of all other chronic conditions. It can also impact a person's quality of life as well as impair social functioning and mental health, and cause bodily pain. It is a costly issue due to a high number of office visits to the healthcare provider, hospital admissions, and medications (both prescription and over-the-counter) to treat the problem, approaching $1 billion annually in the United States (Eoff & Lembro, 2008).

Constipation is difficult or infrequent passage of stool, hardness of stool, or a feeling of incomplete evacuation of the colon with defecation (Merck Manual, 2010). Some elders are concerned with the stool's appearance (size, shape, color) or consistency (soft, hard, or loose). Sometimes the major complaint many people experience is a sense of incomplete evacuation after having a bowel movement (which is also referred to as defecation). Constipation is blamed for many problems, including abdominal pain, nausea, fatigue and anorexia, which may be symptoms of an underlying issue such as irritable bowel syndrome or depression. It is not realistic to expect all symptoms to be relieved by a daily bowel movement, and it should be stressed that medications and treatments to aid bowel habits should be used cautiously. Some elders become obsessive and may feel the need to have a bowel movement daily to rid themselves of "unclean" wastes. Such individuals often spend excessive time on the toilet or become chronic users of laxatives (Merck Manual, 2010).

Constipation may be associated with sluggish movement of stool through the colon. This may be a result of inadequate lower bowel motility. Irritable bowel syndrome (IBS) is a problem with symptoms such as abdominal discomfort and altered bowel habits, but generally normal colonic transit and anorectal functions. Management of IBS is aimed at symptom management. This functional gastrointestinal disorder can manifest primarily as constipation (IBS-C), or diarrhea (IBS-D), or mixed constipation and diarrhea (IBS-M). IBS negatively impacts quality of life for those affected and is associated with significant economic consequences. IBS occurs in 10-20% of the general population and IBS is more common in women than men (Videlock & Chang, 2007; Longstreth, Thompson, Chey, Houghton, Mearin, & Spiller, 2006).

Some elders attempt excessive straining to have a bowel movement because of difficulties due to pelvic floor dysfunctions; this may contribute to issues such as hemorrhoids, anal fissures, and rectal prolapse. Another frequent problem in elderly individuals is fecal impaction, which is hardened stool in the colon that is difficult to evacuate, particularly in those who have decreased mobility. This can also occur after certain diagnostic procedures that use barium (Merck Manual, 2010).

Table 6-1. *Chronic Constipation Definition & Rome III Criteria*	
American College of Gastroenterology Definitions	**Rome III Criteria for Functional Constipation**
Symptom-based disorder defined as unsatisfactory defecation and characterized by infrequent bowel movements, difficult stool passage, or both Difficult stool passage may include: • straining • difficulty passing stool • incomplete evacuation • hard/lumpy stool • prolonged time to defecate or passage of stool • need for manual maneuvers to pass stool Chronic Constipation is defined as the presence of these symptoms for ≥ 3 months	2 or more of the following (criteria must be met in the last 3 months, with symptom onset at least 6 months prior to diagnosis) • straining during at least 25% of defecations • hard or lumpy stools in at least 25% of defecations • sensation of incomplete evacuation in at least 25% of evacuations • manual maneuvers to facilitate at least 25% of defecations • fewer than 3 defecations per week Loose stools are rarely present without the use of laxatives There is insufficient criteria for Irritable Bowel Syndrome (IBS)

(Gallagher, O'Mahony, & Quigley, 2008)

Managing Constipation

Education about constipation, its causes, and ways to manage it is the key to diminishing the problem. Chronic constipation is frequently seen in older adults living in the community, is present in up to 50% of elders in nursing homes/long-term care facilities, and is more prevalent in women (Gallagher, O'Mahony, & Quigley, 2008). According to the American College of Gastroenterology, constipation is a symptom defined as unsatisfactory defecation and is characterized by infrequent bowel movements, difficult stool passage, or both (ACG, 2005). Slow-transit constipation is characterized by prolonged intestinal time (i.e., slow bowel motility), which may be attributable to alterations in the regulation of the enteric nervous system, decreased nitric oxide production, impaired gastrocolic reflex, alterations of neuropeptides, and a reduced number of interstitial cells of Cajal in the colon (Lembo & Camilleri, 2003).

An algorithm for managing chronic constipation was developed to assist in handling this problem. Management begins with a complete history of the problem and a thorough examination to rule out other problems. If any of the following problems are associated with constipation, consider evaluation by a gastrointestinal specialist for further examinations: bleeding, anemia, weight loss, sudden change in stool caliber, and/or abdominal pain.

An initial constipation management algorithm includes:
- increasing fiber in dietary intake
- increasing fluid/water intake
- increasing activity
- incorporating time in an individual's schedule for bowel movements

If these maneuvers fail, then medications are suggested.

Refer for Directed testing

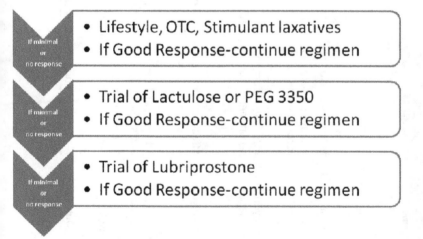

Refer to Specialist

Figure 6-1. *Algorithm to Manage Constipation*

American College of Gastroenterology
Recommendations* for Individuals with Chronic Constipation

	Laxative	Recommendation	Common Side Effects
Bulking Agents	Psyllium (Fiberall, Metamucil)	Increases stool frequency; *Grade B*	Bloating, flatulence, abdominal pain
	Methylcellulose (Citracel, Willpower)	Insufficient data to make a recommendation about efficacy; *Grade B*	Must increase fluid intake with fiber to avoid mechanical obstruction of esophagus and colon
	Polycarbophil (Equalactin, Konsyl Fiber)	Insufficient data to make a recommendation about efficacy; *Grade B*	
Osmotic Laxatives	Magnesium hydroxide (Milk of Magnesia)	Insufficient data to make a recommendation about efficacy; *Grade B*	Flatulence, abdominal cramps, electrolyte abnormalities particularly in patients with renal impairment, cardiac disease
	Polyethylene glycol (Miralax)	Effective at improving stool frequency and stool consistency; *Grade A*	Bitter taste, diarrhea; High doses: diarrhea, nausea, abdominal bloating, cramping, flatulence
	Lactulose (Cephulac, Enulose)	Effective at improving stool frequency and stool consistency; *Grade A*	Bloating, flatulence, Hypokalemia
Stimulant Laxatives	Senna (Senna, Senokot)	Insufficient data to make a recommendation about efficacy; *Grade B*	Abdominal discomfort, cramps, electrolyte imbalance, allergic reactions
	Bisacodyl (Correctal, Dulcolax)	Insufficient data to make a recommendation about efficacy; *Grade B*	

		American College of Gastroenterology Recommendations* for Individuals with Chronic Constipation	
	Laxative	Recommendation	Common Side Effects
Lubricants	Mineral oil	Insufficient data to make a recommendation about efficacy; Grade C	Malabsorption of fat soluble vitamins; lipoid pneumonia if aspirated
	Glycerin suppositories	Not rated	Anorectal irritation
Stool Softeners	Docusate sodium, Docusate calcium (Colace, Dulcolax, Equate, Metamucil)	Insufficient data to make a recommendation about efficacy; may be inferior to psyllium for improvement in stool frequency; **Grade B**	Abdominal cramps, associated with fecal incontinence in elders
Chlorine Channel Activator	Lubiprostone (Amitiza)	Not rated in 2005 review; FDA approved for chronic constipation & IBS-C	Nausea (minimized when taken with food), diarrhea, headache

Grade A: supported by 2 or more level 1 trials, adequate size, appropriate methodology; **Grade B:** based on evidence from a single Level 1 trial or two or more Level 2 trials (inadequate sample sizes and/or inappropriate methodology); **Grade C:** based on non-randomized trials or case studies

Fecal impaction
A fecal impaction is a severe form of constipation in elders; it is a solid, immobile bulk of stool that can develop in the rectum.

Symptoms of Fecal Impaction
- complaints of chronic constipation
- watery stool or fecal incontinence and paradoxical diarrhea as liquid stool passes around the obstruction
- occasionally nausea and/or vomiting secondary to blockage in colon

Causes of fecal impaction
- an older adult who has limited ability to move (such as being bedridden) or persons with severe disease of the nervous system
- taking certain drugs can contribute or cause constipation, including:
  - o Anticholinergic agents, which affect the interaction between certain nerves and muscles
      (Benadryl, Phenergan, Vistaril, Zofran, etc)
  - o Antidiarrhea medications (Immodium, Lomotil, etc)
  - o Narcotic pain medication
  - o Limited water intake
  - o Limited fiber intake

Complications of fecal impaction may include necrosis and ulcers of the rectal tissue, and the hardened stool may cause rupture of the intestine, sepsis, and even death.

Management of Fecal Impactions includes non-invasive treatments similar to those for constipation, such as increased intake of fluids and dietary fiber, and physical exercise. However, once fecal impaction occurs, these methods are usually not effective until the impaction has been removed.

Treatment
Enemas to soften the impaction and manual disimpaction, i.e., digital manipulation by a healthcare practitioner.

Prevention
The following dietary changes can help promote regular, soft, bulky stools:
- Add high-fiber foods to the diet, including whole-wheat grains, fresh vegetables, and beans

- Use products containing psyllium, such as Metamucil, to add bulk to the stools – making sure to add the appropriate amount of water or it can worsen the problem.
- Encourage the individual to drink 2 - 3 liters of fluid a day (unless contraindicated)

(AHQR, 2010; Pare et al, 2007)

BOWEL TRAINING

In some elders, bowel training (or re-training) may be necessary in order to teach the person how to recognize stool in the colon, encourage routine and complete evacuation of stool, and to minimize complications. In certain individuals, digital stimulation to trigger a bowel movement occur may be necessary:

- Insert a lubricated finger into the anus of the individual and make a circular motion until the sphincter relaxes.
- After stimulating the anus, have the person assume a normal posture for a bowel movement.
- If able to walk, have the person sit on the toilet or bedside commode. If the person is confined to the bed, use a bedpan.
- Get the individual as close to a sitting position as possible, or use a left side lying position if the person is unable to sit.
- Try to get as much privacy as possible.
- Reading while sitting on the toilet may help relax someone enough to have a bowel movement.
- If digital stimulation does not produce a bowel movement within 20 minutes, repeat the procedure.
- Ask the individual to try to contract the muscles of the abdomen and bear down while releasing the stool.
- It may be helpful to bend forward while bearing down, which increases abdominal pressure and helps empty the bowel.
- Perform digital stimulation every day until a pattern of regular bowel movements is established.
- Sometimes it may be necessary to stimulate bowel movements by using a suppository (glycerin or Dulcolax) or a small oil enema (Fleets oil enema) for 1 to 2 weeks to train the bowels to move regularly – the recommendation is 3 days a week (for example – on Monday, Wednesday, Friday) for 2 weeks, unless the constipation is severe, then daily may be more appropriate.
- Give the person warm prune juice or fruit nectar to stimulate bowel movements – an old fashioned treatment is a prune juice and coffee combination.

(Med line Plus, 2010)

Consistency is crucial for the success of a bowel retraining program. Establish a set time for daily bowel movements. Choose a time that is convenient, keeping in mind an individual's daily schedule. The best time for a bowel movement is 20 - 40 minutes after a meal because eating generally stimulates bowel activity. Within a few weeks, most people are able to establish a regular routine of bowel movements.

Fecal Incontinence

Fecal incontinence, also referred to as bowel incontinence, is the inability to control bowel movements, causing stool (feces) to leak unexpectedly from a person's rectum. The problem can range from occuring occasionally with leakage of stool while passing gas to a complete loss of bowel control.

Critical to normal bowel function are
- Anal sphincter muscles: external and internal sphincter/muscle control
- Rectal sensation: ability of the body to recognize stool in the colon
- Rectal accommodation: ability to the colon to stretch to contain the stool in the colon

Causes of fecal incontinence
The ability to hold stool requires the normal function of an individual's rectum, anus and nervous system as well as the physical and mental capabilities to recognize and appropriately respond to the urge to defecate. A broad range of conditions and disorders can cause fecal incontinence, including:

Constipation – chronic constipation may lead to a hard, dry stool which is too large to pass, the muscles of the rectum and intestines stretch, and then eventually weaken. Watery stool from above the hardened stool may move around it and leak out. Chronic constipation may also make the nerves of the anus and rectum less responsive to the presence of stool – the individual does not sense the stool in the colon/anal area.

Diarrhea – solid stool is easier to retain in the rectum than is loose stool; loose stools can often lead to fecal incontinence. Liquid diets often result in loose or watery stools.

Muscle damage – injury to the anal sphincter (the rings of muscle at the end of the rectum that help hold the stool in the body); when damaged, they are simply not strong enough to maintain continence and this may allow leakage of stool.

Nerve damage – nerves that control the anal sphincter or those that sense stool in the rectum may become damaged and fecal incontinence can result. Frequent straining to have a bowel movement, spinal cord injury and stroke, as well as diseases that can affect these nerves (such as diabetes and multiple sclerosis), and cause damage leading to fecal incontinence.

Loss of storage capacity (accommodation) in the rectum – the rectum usually stretches to accommodate stool but when the rectum is scarred or rectal walls have stiffened from surgery, radiation treatment or inflammatory bowel disease, such as Crohn's disease or ulcerative colitis, the rectum can't stretch as much as it needs to, so excess stool leaks out.

Surgery – surgery to treat hemorrhoids (enlarged veins in the rectum or anus) can damage the anus and cause fecal incontinence, as can other complex operations involving the rectum and anus.

Rectal cancer – cancers of the anus and rectum may lead to fecal incontinence if the cancer invades the muscle walls or affects the nerve impulses needed for defecation.

Other conditions – if the rectum drops down into the anus (rectal prolapse) or, in women, if the rectum protrudes through the vagina (rectocele), fecal incontinence may result. Hemorrhoids may also prevent complete closure of the anal sphincter, leading to fecal incontinence.

o Loss of muscle strength with age
o Chronic laxative abuse – laxatives can lead to fecal incontinence

(Mayo Clinic, 2010)

Treatment for Fecal Incontinence

Treatment for fecal incontinence can usually help restore bowel control or at least substantially reduce the severity of the condition. Depending upon the cause of the incontinence, treatment may include dietary changes, medications, special exercises, or surgery. IF DIARRHEA IS PRESENT IN AN ELDER, MAKE SURE TO RULE OUT FECAL IMPACTION with watery or loose stools escaping around the hardened mass!

Medications to Manage Fecal Incontinence

Anti-diarrheal drugs – Medications can assist in reducing diarrhea, but are not recommended on a long term basis due to their side effects, as well as the tendency for creating dependence on the medication

- o Loperamide (Imodium) 1 to 2 mg after stools as needed only (every 6 hours); no more than 6 mg daily
- o Diphenoxylate (Lomotil) 1 tab or 2.5 to 5ml after stools as needed (every 6 hours), can interact with MAO inhibitors and cause elevation in blood pressure as well as cause psychosis/delirium in elders – use cautiously in individuals with liver impairment
- o Add bulk to the stools – Metamucil, Konsyl, or Miralax daily: in diarrhea which is chronic – add 1/2 the amount of water suggested to dilute this medication – this encourages the bulking agent to absorb fluid from the intestines
- o Lactobacillus acidophilus (Bacid) can be used if diarrhea occurs after recent use of an antibiotic (or in cases of Irritable Bowel Syndrome with diarrhea predominant) to allow the intestines to build up their natural flora: 1 tablet 3 to 4 times a day for 5 to 14 days (this is also available in powder and liquid form)
- o Laxatives – if chronic constipation is to blame for the fecal incontinence, temporary use of mild laxatives, such as Lactulose or Milk of Magnesia, may help restore normal bowel movements.
- o Stool softeners may be used to prevent stool impaction – Colace, Dulcolax, or Surfax once a day.
- o Other medications – if diarrhea is the cause of the fecal incontinence, consider decreasing the spontaneous motion of the bowels (bowel motility) or medications that decrease the water content of the stool

Managing or Preventing Fecal Incontinence

A variety of therapies may improve fecal incontinence: Dietary changes. What someone eats and drinks affects stool consistency. For example, if chronic constipation is to blame for fecal incontinence, encourage an individual to drink plenty of fluids – especially water, and eat fiber-rich foods that aren't constipating. If diarrhea is contributing to the problem, increase the person's intake of high-fiber foods to add bulk to their stools and make them less watery.

Bowel training. If fecal incontinence is due to a lack of anal sphincter control or decreased awareness of the urge to defecate, a bowel training program and exercise therapies aimed at helping restore muscle strength may be helpful. In some cases, bowel training means learning to go to the toilet at a specific time of day. For example, make a conscious effort to have a bowel movement after eating. This helps someone gain greater control by establishing with some predictability when to have a bowel movement.

Biofeedback is another bowel training treatment for fecal incontinence. It involves inserting a pressure-sensitive probe into the anus. This probe registers muscle strength and activity of the anal sphincter as it contracts around the probe. A person can practice sphincter contractions and learn to strengthen muscles by viewing the scale's display. These exercises can strengthen a person's rectal muscles. (This is especially helpful in individuals who have decreased rectal sensation.)

Treatment for constipation and/or stool impaction. Manual fecal impaction removal may be necessary to evacuate hardened stool (impacted stool) if taking laxatives or using enemas does not help pass the mass of stool. To remove an impacted stool: insert one or two gloved fingers into the rectum to break apart the impacted stool. These smaller pieces are easier to expel.

Sacral nerve stimulation. The sacral nerves run from the spinal cord to muscles in the pelvis. These nerves regulate the sensation and strength of a person's rectal and anal sphincter muscles. Direct electrical stimulation of these nerves can restore bowel continence in 40 to 75 percent of people whose fecal incontinence is caused by nerve damage and whose anal sphincter muscles are intact. This treatment is usually done only if other treatments have not worked. Sacral nerve stimulation is usually carried out in stages. First, four to six small needles are positioned in the muscles of the lower bowel, and these muscles are stimulated by an external pulse generator. The muscle response to the stimulation generally isn't uncomfortable. After a successful response, a permanent pulse generator may be implanted.

Surgery. For some people, treatment of fecal incontinence requires surgery to correct an underlying problem. Surgical procedures to treat fecal incontinence are done only as a last resort. But, certain causes of fecal incontinence – anal sphincter damage caused by childbirth or rectal prolapse, for example – may require surgical intervention.

Colostomy is a surgical procedure which is the ultimate last resort – it is the most definitive way to correct fecal incontinence. It is an operation that diverts stool through an opening in the abdomen. A special bag is attached to this opening to collect the stool.

(Mayo Clinic, 2010)

Chapter 6 References

AHRQ (2010). National Guideline Clearinghouse: Management of Constipation. Retrieved December 26, 2010, from http://www. guideline.gov/content.aspx?id=15434

American College of Gastroenterology Chronic Constipation Task Force. An evidence-based approach to the management of chronic constipation in North America. *American Journal of Gastroenterology.* 2005; 100(S1):1-4.

Eoff, J., & Lembro, A. Optimal treatment of chronic constipation in managed care: review and roundtable discussions. *Managed care Pharm.* 2008: 14(9):S1-S17.

Gallagher P., O'Mahony D., Quigley, E.M. Management of chronic constipation in the elderly. Drugs Aging. 2008;25(10):807-821

Lembo, A., Camilleri, M. Chronic Constipation. *New England Journal of Medicine.* 2003: 349:1360-1368.

Longstreth G., Thompson, W.G., Chey, W.D., Houghton, L.A., Mearin, F., Spiller, R.C. Functional bowel disorders. *Gastroenterology.* 2006;130:1480-1491.

MayoClinic (2010). Abdominal Gas & Bloating. Retrieved December 27, 2010, from http://www.mayoclinic.com/health/gas-and-gas-pains/ DS00080

Merck Manual (2010). Constipation. Retrieved December 24, 2010, from http://www.merckmanuals.com/professional/sec02/ch008/ch008b. html?qt=defecation&alt=sh

Merck Manual of Geriatrics (2010). Gastrointestinal Issues. Retrieved December 26, 2010, from http://www.merckmanuals.com/ professional/sec02/ch008/ch008a.html

Paré, P., Bridges, R., Champion, M., Ganguli, S., Gray, J., Irvine E., Plourde, V., Poitras, P., Turnbull, G., Moayyedi, P., Flook, N., & Collins, S. (2007). Recommendations on chronic constipation (including constipation associated with irritable bowel syndrome) treatment. *Canadian Journal of Gastroenterology.* Apr21 Suppl B:3B-22B.

Videlock, E., Chang, L. Irritable bowel syndrome: current approach to symptoms, evaluation, and treatment. *Gastroenterol Clinics of North America.* 2007;36:66

Urinary Incontinence

Older adults have many changes affecting their ability to hold their urine, which can lead to urinary incontinence. This problem can be embarrassing and cause depression, anxiety, and social isolation in many elders. This chapter will discuss the causes of urinary incontinence and ways to diminish the problem.

Urinary Incontinence – A Major Problem in Elders

Urinary incontinence is a worrisome problem in older individuals and can lead to infections, decreased quality of life, depression, and social isolation from fear of other people noticing the urinary incontinence. This issue impacts physical functioning, may cause psychological distress, and is costly due to use of medications and incontinence pads. There are many changes that occur with normal aging that predispose an older person to issues of urinary incontinence.

Renal & Urinary System

All aspects of the functioning of a person's kidneys are affected by age. By the age of 80, an individual will have a 50% reduction in the number of nephrons and the kidneys will decrease by at least 50% in their ability to filter fluid and the waste products of the body (Urinary System, 2007). The kidney is less efficient in removing medications from the bloodstream, which may allow a build-up of blood levels of a medication.

Aging changes to Kidneys:

- The size and function of the kidneys will diminish in direct correlation to size and weight of the other organs of the body.
- There is loss of glomeruli and the kidneys become stiffer and sclerotic.
- Arteriosclerosis affects the blood vessels that supply the urinary system.
- The large renal vessels show sclerosis but no reduction in the vessel lumen is seen.

- Blood flow through the kidneys decreases from 1200 ml/min to an average of 600 ml/min as a result of fixed anatomic and structural changes.
- The Glomerular Filtration Rate (GFR) steadily declines and is measured by creatinine clearance, which is directly related to muscle mass and is a product of muscle metabolism. By 80 years of age, the Creatinine clearance is decreased to 100 ml/min. Approximately 1/3 of elders do not exhibit a decline in GFR. Plasma Creatinine clearance is constant throughout all ages and a decline in urine Creatinine clearance is an important indicator of appropriate drug therapy in an older adult. A random serum Creatinine may not be truly reflective of kidney function in some elders due to changes in lean muscle mass – GFR and 24-hour urine tests for Creatinine clearance are more accurate in assessing kidney function (Crum, 2008).
- Basal renin is reduced in aging kidneys with a parallel reduction in aldosterone. This can decrease an older individual's ability to conserve sodium and cause a slight shift in the antidiuretic hormone (ADH), further reducing the body's ability to concentrate urine and conserve water.
- Under normal circumstances, kidney function should be sufficient to meet the regulation and excretion demands of the body, but when there is poor circulation, stress of disease, surgery, or fever, there is reduced ability to respond, as well as decreased ability to recover

(Ebersole et al, 2004).

Urinary System Changes in the Elderly Individual

The Urinary Bladder is a reservoir for filtered fluids and waste products of the body. In aging individuals, the bladder tissue becomes much less elastic or stretchable, decreasing the amount of urine the bladder is able to hold. The muscles of the bladder also become weaker, making emptying the bladder less efficient and allowing urine to remain in the bladder after voiding (Aging Changes of the Urinary System, 2009). The sensation of the need to urinate can be delayed in many older individuals due to decreased ability of the body to interpret the nerve sensation of a full bladder. Thus the need to urinate may be sudden and urgent.

The pelvic floor muscles commonly get weaker with age in both sexes. In women, childbirth may contribute to this weakness, as well as normal changes due to menopause – estrogen assists in strengthening the pelvic muscles and after menopause there is a lack of estrogen and thus a slightly diminished muscle tone in the pelvic region. Pelvic muscles may become so weak that the bladder and urethra prolapse, or drop into the vagina resulting in an older female becoming incontinent, or to lose urine involuntarily. The normal delay in feeling the urge to urinate adds to this problem to make incontinence quite common in older women.

In men, urine flow can be blocked by an enlarged prostate gland, known as benign prostatic hyperplasia or BPH. The prostate lies just below the bladder and surrounds part of the urethra. BPH may cause difficulty starting the urine stream, a weak urine stream and dribbling of urine, and lead to incomplete voiding of urine from the bladder (Rajaratnam, 2009).

Urinary Incontinence

Urinary incontinence is the involuntary loss of urine significant enough to be bothersome (Castronova, 2007). It can be an embarrassing problem and can cause a multitude other problems, including skin irritation, skin breakdown, and infections. It has been estimated that up to 2/3 of all older adults experience this problem, which can lead to other issues such as urinary tract infections and depression (Lippincott, 2009). The severity of urinary incontinence ranges from occasionally leaking urine with stress, such as coughing or sneezing, to having a sudden and strong urge to urinate, causing incontinence before an individual is able to make it to a place to void (also known as urinating or empty the bladder). Urinary incontinence can affect a person's day-to-day activities, diminish quality of life, cause isolation, and lead to depression, as well as increase other behavioral problems in confused elders, such as agitation and aggression. It is a costly problem in elders, especially those in the Nursing Home setting, due to the high cost of disposable pads/diapers, staff costs to change a wet individual, and the high use of agents to manage anxiety and behavioral problems in incontinent elders. There are some simple lifestyle changes and medical treatments which can ease discomfort, improve the problem, or stop urinary incontinence.

Bladder Functioning

Normal bladder function consists of 2 phases: filling & emptying. The normal micturition cycle, which is storage of urine and voiding (emptying of the bladder), requires the bladder and the urethral sphincter to work together as a coordinated unit. During storage of urine, the bladder acts as a low-pressure receptacle and the urinary sphincter maintains resistance to prevent the flow of urine. During the urine elimination phase, the bladder contracts to void while the urinary sphincter opens (low resistance) to allow unobstructed urinary flow and bladder emptying (Ebersole et al, 2004). Elders can experience problems with urinary incontinence, but there are many types of urinary incontinence and there ARE ways to treat the problem and improve quality of life for our incontinent elders.

Types of urinary incontinence and common causes

Stress incontinence is the loss of urine due to stress of pressure in the abdominal area from causes such as coughing, sneezing, laughing, exercising or lifting something heavy. This type of urinary incontinence occurs when the sphincter muscle of the bladder is weakened.

Urge incontinence is a sudden, intense urge to urinate, followed by involuntary loss of urine. The bladder muscle contracts, giving a warning of only a few seconds to a minute to allow a person to reach a place to urinate or to reach a toilet. With urge incontinence, the need to urinate occurs frequently, including throughout the night-time. Urge incontinence may be caused by urinary tract infections, bladder irritants, bowel problems, Parkinson's disease, Alzheimer's disease, stroke, injury or nervous system damage associated with multiple sclerosis. May also be referred to as an overactive bladder.

Overflow incontinence is frequent or constant dribbling of urine; it is an inability to empty the bladder effectively. Some individuals may produce a weak stream of urine. This type of urinary incontinence can be caused by a damaged bladder, blocked urethra or nerve damage from diabetes and, in men, it can be caused by an enlarged prostate gland.

Mixed incontinence is a combination of stress incontinence and urge incontinence

Functional incontinence is incontinence of urine caused by a physical problem which affects a person's mobility (arthritis or stroke) or a psychological issue such as mental impairment, that keeps an individual from making it to the toilet in time.

Gross total incontinence is a continuous leaking of urine, day and night, or the periodic uncontrollable leaking of large volumes of urine due to the bladder having no storage capacity. This type of incontinence can be due to a congenital anatomical defect, injuries to the spinal cord or urinary system, or by a fistula between the bladder and an adjacent structure, such as the vagina (Urinary Incontinence, Mayo Clinic 2010).

Common causes of temporary urinary incontinence
Certain foods, drinks and medications can cause temporary urinary incontinence. A simple change in habits can bring relief.

Overhydration – drinking a lot of fluids over a short period of time, which can suddenly increase the amount of urine.
Dehydration – when an individual does not consume enough liquid to stay hydrated, the urine can occasionally become very concentrated, which can irritate the bladder and lead to or worsen urinary incontinence.

Caffeine is a diuretic and can stimulant the bladder, leading to a sudden need to urinate. Caffeine is found in many beverages (soft drinks, coffee, and tea) and foods (chocolate and certain ice creams).

Bladder irritation – many other substances can aggravate an individual's bladder, including carbonated drinks, tea and coffee – with or without caffeine, artificial sweeteners, corn syrup, and foods and beverages that are high in spice, sugar and acid, such as citrus and tomatoes.

Medications – certain medications can affect a person's production of urine as well as the ability to urinate: heart medications, blood pressure drugs, sedatives, muscle relaxants and others

Treatable medical conditions which may be responsible for urinary incontinence

Urinary tract infections (UTIs) can irritate the bladder, causing a strong urge to urinate and can lead to or worsen urinary incontinence. Other possible signs and symptoms of a UTI include a burning sensation when urinating, frequent urination, urinating through-out the night (nocturia), urinary urgency, foul-smelling urine, and possibly back pain.

Constipation – Since the rectum is located near the bladder and shares many of the same nerves. Hard, compacted stool in an individual's rectum can cause these nerves to be overactive and increase urinary frequency – possibly leading to urinary incontinence.

Bladder changes with aging and ways to manage
      Aging of the bladder muscle leads to a decrease in the bladder's capacity to store urine and an increase in overactive bladder symptoms. In women, after menopause – the female organs may atrophy (diminish in size) or be absent (if surgically removed) and there is more space in the abdominal cavity. And this, in combination with slightly weaker abdominal muscles, can allow a woman to empty the bladder incompletely, which can allow stagnation of a small amount of urine. In men, the prostate increases in size and may present a blockage to emptying the bladder. And in combination with increased abdominal girth, this may increase the difficulty of a man to completely empty his bladder.

There are many lifestyle factors which affect urination, including chronic medical conditions, use of certain medications, increased weight, and a variety of other factors. Certain lifestyle changes (such as stopping smoking, treating high blood pressure, and keeping weight within a healthy range) can help curb symptoms of an overactive bladder and thus improve urination and decrease urinary incontinence. The following are medical conditions which can lead to urinary incontinence:

Prostatitis is inflammation of the prostate gland in males. Although loss of bladder control in males is not a typical sign of prostatitis, urinary incontinence sometimes occurs with this problem. Symptoms may include pain in the scrotal or rectal area, urinary frequency, urinary hesitancy, nocturia, blood in urine, or bacteria in urine. Prostatitis is often managed by increasing water intake, wearing loose fitting underwear, minimizing sitting (causing pressure on the prostate) and, in certain individuals, with an antibiotic medication.

Enlarged Prostate or Prostate cancer – Stress incontinence, or urge incontinence, can be associated with untreated prostate enlargement, as well as with prostate cancer. However, incontinence is a side effect of treatments – surgery or radiation – for prostate cancer. All men should have an annual prostate examination after the age of 40. And any male who has complaints of urinary hesitancy, urinary incontinence, and an increase in nocturia warrants examination by a healthcare practitioner (AHRQ, 2010).

Bladder cancer or bladder stones – Incontinence, urinary urgency and burning with urination can be signs and symptoms of bladder cancer or bladder stones. Other signs and symptoms include blood in the urine and pelvic or lower abdominal pain.

Neurological disorders such as Multiple Sclerosis, Parkinson's disease, stroke, a brain tumor or a spinal injury can interfere with nerve signals involved in bladder control, causing urinary incontinence.

Obstruction – A tumor anywhere along the urinary tract can obstruct the normal flow of urine and cause incontinence, usually overflow incontinence. Urinary stones – hard, stone-like masses that can form in the bladder – may be to blame for urine leakage. Stones can be present in the kidney, bladder or ureter.

Complications of urinary incontinence include:

Skin problems – Urinary incontinence can lead to rashes, fungal dermatitis, skin infections, and sores (skin ulcers) from constantly wet skin.

Urinary tract infections – Incontinence increases an elder's risk of urinary tract infections.

Changes in activities – Urinary incontinence may keep an elder from participating in normal activities. Some individuals may stop exercising, quit attending social gatherings or even stop venturing away from familiar areas to places where toilets may be difficult to find/access.

Changes in personal life – Incontinence can have a negative impact on an elder's personal life. It's not uncommon for an incontinent person to experience anxiety, depression, and agitation/behavioral problems.

Managing Urinary Incontinence

Urinary incontinence is a worrisome issue for many elders and warrants management to improve quality of life for an elder, as well as to prevent complications. Simple management techniques include:

Scheduled toileting – schedule voiding or trips to the restroom/ toilet every 2 to 4 hours or according to an individual's toilet habits.

Prompted voiding – check for dryness and encourage use of the toilet; have the person at least make an effort to sit on the toilet and attempt to void.

Improved access to toilets – use equipment to assist the elder to ambulate to the toilet independently, if possible, with such devices as canes, walkers, wheelchairs; also consider devices that raise the seating level of toilets to make toileting easier.

Managing fluids and diet – eliminate dietary caffeine (for those with urge incontinence), encourage water intake throughout the day (but limit fluid intake 2-3 hours before bedtime), and encourage adequate fiber in the diet.

Disposable absorbent garments – use these, if necessary, to keep an individual dry.

Techniques to decrease Urinary Incontinence
Behavioral techniques and lifestyle changes, as well as muscle strengthening, will work well for certain types of urinary incontinence. Some of these techniques may be the only treatment needed.

To strengthen pelvic muscles of a woman – Kegel exercises:

- **Find the right muscles**. To locate the muscles which make the bladder hold urine when stressed: attempt to stop the stream of urine or an individual may insert a finger inside the vaginal entrance and try to squeeze the surrounding muscles. Then relax the muscles.
- **Perfect the technique**. Once an individual has identified the pelvic floor muscles that assist in voiding, an individual should empty their bladder and sit or lie down. Contract the pelvic floor muscles, hold the contraction for five seconds, then relax for five seconds. Try it four or five times in a row. Work up to keeping the muscles contracted for 10 seconds at a time, relaxing for 10 seconds between contractions.
- **Maintain focus**. For best results, focus on tightening only the pelvic floor muscles. Be careful not to flex the muscles in the abdomen, thighs or buttocks. An individual should be encouraged to avoid holding their breath. Rather, a person should breathe freely during the exercises.

- Repeat three times a day. Aim for at least three sets of 10 repetitions each day.

Bladder training – to increase the capacity of the bladder: delaying urination after feeling the urge to void – wait 10 minutes every time an individual feels the urge to void, to lengthen the time between trips to urinate to every two to four hours.

Double voiding – urinating, then waiting a few minutes & urinating again. Women may also find it helpful to lean forward and press on the lower abdomen while voiding to assist in completely emptying the bladder. This will help an individual empty his/her bladder more completely and avoid overflow incontinence. To assist in controlling urges to urinate: When an individual feels the urge to urinate, relax – breathe slowly and deeply – or distract the person with an activity.

Scheduled toileting or timed toileting – toilet according to a schedule rather than waiting for the need to go; schedule toilet visits every two to four hours.

Fluid and diet management – cut back on or avoid alcohol, caffeine or acidic foods. Reduce liquid consumption, lose weight or increase physical activity. Caution must be taken for elders to drink an adequate amount of water to prevent dehydration and urinary tract infections.

Physical therapy
- Pelvic floor muscle exercises to strengthen the urinary sphincter and pelvic floor muscles – the muscles that help control urination.
- Kegels: stop the urine flow, squeeze the muscles used to stop urinating and hold for a count of three and repeat (as described above).
- Electrical stimulation. A procedure in which electrodes are temporarily inserted into the rectum or vagina to stimulate and strengthen pelvic floor muscles. Gentle electrical stimulation can be effective for stress incontinence and urge incontinence, but it takes several months and multiple treatments for this method to work.

Medications
Anticholinergics are indicated for the treatment of overactive bladder with symptoms of urge urinary incontinence, urgency, and frequency. They should be used cautiously in older individuals due to the potential side effects of increasing confusion, falls, constipation, and urinary hesitancy. The preference is for once a day dosing at bedtime:

- oxybutynin (Ditropan) 5 to 10 mg once or twice a day
  - also available in extended release form – Ditropan XL
- olterodine (Detrol) 1 to 2 mg once or twice a day
- darifenacin (Enablex) 7.5 to 15 mg once a day
- solifenacin (VESIcare) 5 to 10 mg daily
- trospium (Sanctura) 20 mg once or twice a day

Another Issue affecting Urination
A Neurogenic Bladder is a malfunctioning urinary bladder due to neurologic dysfunction or insult caused by internal or external trauma, disease, or injury. A neurogenic bladder can cause incomplete emptying of the bladder and the individual may be unable to empty the bladder (also known as urinary retention). This issue is managed with either periodic catherization of a person's bladder or by inserting an indwelling urinary catheter.

Other Urinary Complaints in Elders
There are other urinary complaints common among elders, including dysuria (burning sensations with urination), which is a very irritating problem. Cystitis is the medical term for inflammation of the bladder. Frequently, this inflammation is caused by a bacterial infection; in which case, it may be referred to as a urinary tract infection (UTI). A bladder infection can be painful and bothersome, and can become a serious health problem if the infection spreads to a person's kidneys. Less commonly, cystitis may occur as a reaction to certain drugs, radiation therapy or potential irritants, such as feminine hygiene spray, powders and lotions, or long-term use of a catheter.

Cystitis symptoms
- A strong, persistent urge to urinate
- A burning sensation when urinating
- Passing frequent, small amounts of urine
- Blood in the urine (hematuria)
- Passing cloudy or strong-smelling urine
- Discomfort in the pelvic area
- A feeling of pressure in the lower abdomen
- Low-grade fever

Mayo Clinic (2010)

Bacterial cystitis Bacteria can enter the urinary tract through the urethra and may begin to multiply. The urinary system is designed to prevent bacteria build up in the bladder: the bladder secretes a protective coating that prevents bacteria from attaching to its wall and urine has antibacterial properties that inhibit the growth of bacteria. However, certain factors can lead to increased abnormal bacterial growth (antibiotic use can cause the destruction of a person's 'good' bacteria and allow abnormal/problematic bacteria to grow, which can lead to fungal infections). A bacterial UTI can cause a person's kidney to become infected and cause sepsis in an elder who is susceptible or is frail. Many elders will have bacteria present in their urine but may not exhibit symptoms of an infection (Kamel, 2005). become infected and cause sepsis in an elder who is susceptible or is frail. Many elders will have bacteria present in their urine but may not exhibit symptoms of an infection (Kamel, 2005).

Bacteria in the urine without symptoms, known as Asymptomatic Bacteriuria is characterized by a bacterial count in the urine absent of symptoms such as dysuria, urinary frequency, incontinence of recent onset, flank pain, fever, or other signs of infection. 10-20% of elders have asymptomatic bacteruria and as high as 40-50% of elders in the Nursing Home setting have this issue. Asymptomatic means the elder does not have any new complaints new or different complaints of urinary problems but have a large prescence of bacteria in a single sample of urine. Only 30% of asymptomatic elders have a true urinary tract infection and require treatment with antibiotics.. Management may be aimed at increasing water intake (unless there is a contraindication) and use of an antibiotic medication may not be necessary unless the individual has a history of nephritis (kidney infection or sepsis related to UTIs). Other circumstances which require treatment with an antibiotic include individuals who plan to have hip replacement, individuals who plan to have surgery on their prostate, and those elders who have a history of sepsis due to frequent urinary tract infections.

Sporadic infections are defined as more than 3 episodes of asymptomatic bacteriuria within 1 year. Recurrent infections are classified as either relapse or re-infection UTI. Relapse UTI is an infection in which urine is rendered partially or temporarily sterile by antimicrobial therapy, with the subsequent recurrence of bacteriuria from the uneradicated pathogen, generally within 2 weeks of completion of therapy. Re-infection UTI is defined as an infection that arises more than 4 weeks after the previous infection has been cured; the bacterial strain is often different from the strain that caused the successfully-treated previous infection.

Treatment for a symptomatic UTI should begin with increasing water intake. Urinary symptoms that do not resolve with increasing water intake and eliminating soft drinks, coffee, and tea may require medication management. There is a diversity of potential different types of bacteria, often making it necessary to obtain urine cultures in elderly persons with suspected UTI. Often a Urinalysis, as well as checking a urine culture and sensitivity to specific antibiotics, may be indicated to assure the proper medication is used (Kamel, 2005). Treatment should not be delayed while waiting for culture and sensitivity results. Some clinicians start empiric treatment based on previous culture and sensitivity results, as well as information of a sensitivity pattern in a community or at a facility.

Asymptomatic bacteriuria does not always need to be treated with a medication BUT, if necessary – use these general guidelines. Many organisms (especially E.Coli) which cause urinary tract infections often lose their virulence and become susceptible to the bactericidal effect of normal human plasma. If treatment is necessary, there are certain guidelines to follow in elders. Most elderly women with uncomplicated lower tract UTI should be treated with antibiotics for 10 days; elderly men are generally treated for 14 days. Abbreviated courses (less than 7 days) or treatment for UTI are not recommended for elderly patients, because of relatively high rates of failure and relapse. Older individuals with pyelonephritis or urosepsis should be treated a minimum of 14 days. Intravenous antibiotics may be given if the patient is not able to take antibiotics orally because of vomiting (Kamel, 2005).

TO TREAT OR NOT TO TREAT *a Urinary Tract Infection in an Older Adult*
In order to meet the criteria for treatment of a suspected UTI without an indwelling urinary catheter, 3 symptoms for 3 days – increase water intake – then, if necessary, treat with an antibiotic medication. 3 of the following should be met:
- Fever (> 38°C) or chills
- New or increased burning pain on urination
- New flank or suprapubic pain or tenderness
- Changes in character of urine
- Worsening mental function

Criteria for a suspected UTI with an indwelling urinary catheter; 2 of the following should be met:
- Fever (> 38°C) or chills
- New flank or suprapubic pain or tenderness
- Changes in character of urine
- Worsening mental function

(Kamel, 2005)

Commonly used Antibiotics for UTIs in Elders

- doxycycline (Doxy or Vibra Tab) 100 mg twice a day for 10 days
- ciprofloxin (Cipro) 500 mg twice a day for 10 days
- nitrofuratin (Macrobid) 100 mg twice a day for 10 days
- sulfamethoxazole and trimethoprim (Bactrim DS) twice a day for 7-10 days
- levofloxacin (Levaquin) 250 mg once a day for 10 days
- ceftriaxone (Rocephin) injectable (500 to 1000 mg) intramuscular one time dose or daily for 3 days

*for fungal infections – fluconazole (Diflucan) 100 mg once daily for 3 to 10 days OR Nystatin cream to external genitalia twice a day for 2 weeks

Chapter 7 References

Aging Changes in the Urinary System (2009). Retrieved May 16, 2009, from http://www.drrajmd.com/resources/education/aging_changes_in_the_urinary_sys.htm

AHRQ (2010). Screening for prostate cancer: Clinical summary of a U.S. Preventive Services Task Force Recommendation. Retrieved December 28, 2010, from http://www.annals.org/content/149/3/185.full

Castronovo, A. (2007). Urinary Incontinence in Older Adults Part 1-Transient Urinary Incontinence. Try This: Best Practices in Nursing Care to older Adults. Hartford Institute for Geriatric Nursing. New York University. 11.1

Crum, K. (2008). Creatinine levels in the elderly. Clinical Advisor. Retrieved December 27, 2010, from http://www.clinicaladvisor.com/creatinine-levels-in-the-elderly/article/121835

Ebersole, Hess, & Luggen (2004). Toward Healthy Aging. 6th ed

Kamel, H. (2010). Managing Urinary Tract Infections in the Nursing Home: Myths, Mysteries and Realities. The Internet Journal of Geriatrics and Gerontology. Retrieved April 26, 2010, from http://www.ispub.com/ostia/index.php?xmlFilePath=journals/ijgg/vol1n2/uri.xml

Kamel, H. (2005). Managing Urinary Tract Infections: Guide for Nursing Home Practitioners. Annals of Long Term Care. 13(9).

Lippincott's Nursing Center. (2009). How to Try This: The Assessment of Transient Urinary Incontinence in Older Adults. Retrieved January 13, 2010, from http://www.nursingcenter.com/prodev/ce_article.asp?tid=843349

Mayo Clinic. (2010). Cystitis. Retrieved January 16, 2010, from http://www.mayoclinic.com/health/cystitis/DS00285

Mayo Clinic (2010). Urinary Incontinence. Retrieved March 22, 2010, from http://www.mayoclinic.com/health/urinary-incontinence/DS00404/DSECTION=treatments-and-drugs

Merck Manual. (2010). UTI. Retrieved April 26, 2010, from http://www.merck.com/mkgr/mmg/sec12/ch100/ch100a.jsp

Rackley, R., Vasavada, S., Firoozi, F., & Ingber, M. (2009). Neurogenic Bladder: eMedicine WebMD. Retrieved January 26, 2010, from http://emedicine.medscape.com/article/453539-overview

Rajaratnam, E. (2009). Aging changes in the urinary system. Retrieved May 16, 2009, from http://www.drrajmd.com/resources/education/aging_changes_in_the_urinary_sys.htm

Urinary Incontinence. (2010). Retrieved January 26, 2010, from http://www.bing.com/health/article/mayo-117583/Urinary-incontinence?q=urinary+incontinence&FORM=K1RE

Urinary System. (2007). TLC Nursing Continuing Education Units. Retrieved May 16, 2009, from http://www.tlcnursingceus.com/tlc-courses/urinary-system.htm

Chapter 8
Anxiety & Cognition

Elders can experience anxiety and irritability due to constipation, infections, depression, cognition impairment, and a variety of other causes. Cognitive decline and dementia (including Alzheimer's disease) are not normal changes in the elderly population but do occur. This chapter will present common presentations of anxious elders, cognition issues (including the various dementias), and ways to troubleshoot and manage these problems.

One's quickness of thinking normally slows as an individual ages, but a person's thinking processes are not generally affected. It may take longer to respond, but the ability to respond is still intact in most elders. After the age of 20, people begin to lose brain cells a few at a time and a person's body starts to make fewer of the chemicals the brain cells need to work as efficiently. As individuals age, thinking processes slow slightly and these chemical changes affect memory to some degree. Aging will affect one's memory by changing the way the brain stores information and making it harder for older adults to recall stored information (FamilyDoctor, 2010).

After the age of 60, individuals experience some degree of neuron loss in their brains, mainly in the brain and spinal cord and most pronounced in cerebral cortex. This will cause the size and weight of the brain to diminish slightly (Medline Plus, 2010; Alzheimer's disease Research, 2010). Neuronal dendrites atrophy with aging, which causes an impairment of the synapses and changes in transmission by the chemical neurotransmitters. Growing older means there will be some atrophy within a person's brain and some changes within the workings of the brain, but these changes generally do not affect the brain's functioning – including the ability to reason and remember.

Aging changes do not generally affect the ability of the brain to think, to reason, and to store new memories, unless there is a pathological condition causing a problem. In older adults, the quickness of thinking may slow, but the *ability* to think is not affected under normal circumstances.

Confusion, anxiety, and depression are not normal in older individuals. Some causes of confusion or changes in cognition include illness and medications. There are some conditions which can cause mental health problems in aging individuals, such as dementia (including dementia of Alzheimer's disease) and depression. The main goal of care for elders experiencing problems in their ability to think and remember is to determine the cause of the confusion in order to determine the appropriate treatment. Sometimes there is a reversible factor which can be addressed and the confusion is resolved. Any older person who has problems with memory should undergo a full medical work-up to rule out treatable causes, obtain an accurate diagnosis, and an appropriate plan of care created to meet that person's unique needs.

Issues affecting the Mental Health of Older Adults

Anxiety, depression, and dementia can be problematic in elders, reduce quality of life, be difficult to diagnose and differentiate, and are costly to manage. But these conditions are not a normal part of aging. Often complicating the issue is the fact that many older individuals have multiple medical conditions, many physical problems, and use a number of prescription medications that can lead to anxiety and/ or depression. All of these can combine to lead to anxiety symptoms in the older adult (AMHC, 2007). It must be realized that diagnosing anxiety in individuals with dementia is more difficult: agitation typical of dementia may be confused with anxiety; impaired memory may be interpreted as a sign of anxiety or dementia, and fear may be exacerbate anxiety in a confused elder.

Recognizing anxiety in elders – Observe for any newly-developed problems:

1. Apathy or a loss of interest in activities an individual once enjoyed
2. New fears, as well as loss of confidence, are often triggered by an event such as a fall or other debilitating health condition
3. Often becomes restless or irritable
4. Avoids social situations
5. Changes in daily routine or habits, or becoming secluded in one's home
6. Consider any excessive worries, particularly if they seem to occur more fequently or are out of proportion to reality
7. Trouble sleeping – sleeping too much or too little
8. Other physical symptoms, such as chest pains, palpitations or shortness of breath

Anxiety may be a symptom of another problem in elders. The presentation may range from mild apprehension to a disabling problem.

Causes of Anxiety:
- Urinary tract infection (UTI)
- Upper respiratory infection (URI)
- Constipation
- Dehydration
- Hypothyroidism
- Depression
- Endocrine or other neurological problem
- Medications (over-the-counter, as well as prescription)
  - o antidepressants with stimulating properties, or caffeine, can cause or exacerbate anxiety

Memory & Cognitive Impairments (Dementia)

After the age of 60, individuals experience some degree of neuron loss in their brains, causing the size and weight of the brain to diminish slightly (Alzheimer's disease Research, 2010). But this does not affect the ability of the brain to think, to reason, and to store new memories unless a pathological condition is causing a problem. Essentially, the quickness of thinking may slow as one ages, but the ability to think does not change. Most older individuals are able to think, function, live independently, and manage everyday activities throughout their lives. The main goal of care for elders experiencing problems in their ability to think and remember is to determine the cause of the confusion in order to manage it appropriately.

Causes of Memory Loss & Anxiety in Older Individuals

- Head Trauma
- Nutritional deficiencies (including anemia)
- Neurodegenerative diseases
- Thyroid disease
- Cardiac Arrhythmias (heart-rate abnormalities)
- Seizures
- Strokes or Transient Ischemic Attacks (TIAs)
- Electroconvulsive Therapy
- Infections/Illness
  o Urinary Tract Infections
  o Upper Respiratory Infections
- Dehydration
- Depression
- Medications
  o Benzodiazepines, Barbituates, etc.
- Alcohol Abuse
- Dementia (Alzheimer's disease & other dementias)

Medical Work-up for Elders Presenting with Anxiety or Confusion

Any older person who presents with confusion should undergo a full medical workup, including a physical examination, laboratory tests, and other diagnostic tests as determined necessary by the healthcare provider. All of these tests are helpful in ruling out other problems, which are potentially reversible, and determining an accurate diagnosis. To assist in diagnosing the problem, practitioners should conduct an in-depth history of the elder's day-to-day functioning and any problems in behavior. It is important to obtain as much information as possible from the person, first-hand. But it is also essential to obtain additional information from family and friends who may observe behaviors – this will provide a more reliable picture of the person and of the issues.

Table 8-1. *Potential laboratory work-up for confusion*	
Laboratory test	**Rationale**
CBC	*anemia or infection*
Vit B 12	*anemia*
Homocystine	*anemia*
C reactive protein	*inflammatory process*
Thyroid functioning	*Hypothyroidism*
Liver functioning	*Liver disease/Metabolic disease*
Renal functioning	*Uremia/Kidney disease*
Electrolytes/serum calcium	*Electrolyte disturbances*
Glucose	*Hypo or Hyperglycemia/Diabetes*
Lipid panel	*Hypercholesterolemia*
Baseline EKG	*Slow or Fast Heart-rate*
RPR	*Syphilis*

Diagnostic tests for Elders with Confusion/Memory Issues
1. CT scan of the head
   - Changes due to later stages of Alzheimer's disease (AD)
   - Reduction in size of the brain
2. Magnetic Resonance Imaging (MRI)
   - To rule out other causes such as Cerebrovascular Accident (CVA), Strokes, or tumors
   - May see structural changes associated with Alzheimer's disease
3. PET or SPECT scanning
   - Difference in brain activity between normal brain & Alzheimer's disease (AD)
   - Can help differentiate AD from other forms of dementia
4. Other
   - Neuropsychiatric testing (if appropriate)
   - Central Spinal Fluid analysis (if meningitis is suspected)

Depression

Depression can present as anxiety and be confused with dementia in older individuals. Sometimes people over the age of 60 are treated as if they have dementia when they become forgetful or present with symptoms of self-neglect: does not eat right, does not pay attention to personal hygiene, or have issues sleeping – too much or too little, or exhibit behavioral problems. Elders can have many reasons to be depressed depending on their circumstances: many have chronic medical conditions and experience chronic pain or fatigue; many medications can cause an older person to feel bad; many have lost their loved ones and outlived their friends; and some have lost their homes due to inability to live independently and have been placed in a nursing home setting. But being sad and sedentary is not an expectation of mood and level of functioning for people as they age. Depression is often under-diagnosed and under-treated in the older population.

Table 8-2. *Symptoms of Depression*	
Sad or Depressed Symptoms	**Anxious Symptoms**
No interest or pleasure in things one used to enjoy, including sex	Anxiety
	Restlessness
Feeling sad or numb	Chronic complaints, i.e., pain, constipation, insomnia, etc.
Crying easily or for no reason	
Feeling slowed down	Muscle irritability
Feeling worthless or guilty	Irritability
Change in appetite; unintended change in weight	Concentration problems
	Headaches, backaches or digestive problems
Trouble recalling things, concentrating or making decisions	Insomnia
Problems sleeping, or wanting to sleep all of the time	
Feeling tired all of the time	
Thoughts about death or suicide	

Depression can lead to physical and psychological impairment, as well as diminish quality of life. Older adults who are depressed and do not take care themselves, or of their medical conditions, will likely experience a decline in overall health. For example: an individual with a diagnosis of heart failure who does not adhere to a low salt diet, does not take his diuretic medication, and leads a sedentary lifestyle – the heart failure will worsen and the person will become sicker. Or if a diabetic person takes insulin and does not eat appropriately – the person's glucose level drops and possibly leads to a hypoglycemia episode.

Self-neglect due to depression worsens an older person's overall health and diminishes quality of life. Depression can cause worsening of chronic medical conditions in elders, lead to increased healthcare costs, and increase the costs of healthcare for society, since many of these elders end up in an acute care hospital where management is quite costly. Individuals who are not capable of caring, or not willing to care, for their medical issues often end up in a long term care setting such as a Nursing Home, where costs for care are expensive. Depression can also lead to suicide in elders. For example, an obese male with a history of congestive heart failures ingests a month's worth of cardiac medications over a short period of time or he does not take any of his medications at all. Care must be taken to appropriately diagnose depression and treat the problem to lessen the occurrence of such problems.

Dementia

A person who has a dementia may have an altered perception of reality, due to the disease. Each day brings different behaviors and new demands, and may present opportunities as the caregiver copes with a person's changing levels of ability. Abrupt changes in behavior may pose a greater challenge to management than cognitive decline for individuals with dementia and their caregivers. The nature and frequency of problematic behaviors varies over the course of an illness, but in most individuals, these symptoms occur more often in the later stages of disease (Rayner et al, 2006).

Management of individuals with a diagnosis of dementia requires a comprehensive approach that incorporates a combination of strategies. It begins with an accurate assessment of symptoms, awareness of the environment in which symptoms occur, and identification of factors that precipitate symptoms, as well as noting how the symptoms affect individuals and their caregivers. Non-pharmacologic interventions are the foundation of care and include creating a simplistic and safe environment, a predictable routine, counseling for caregivers about the unintentional nature of psychotic symptoms, and offering strategies to manage and cope with troubling behaviors. Approaches to diminish the occurrence of problematic behaviors involve a structured environment, behavior modification, appropriate use of sensory intervention, and maintenance of routines, such as providing meals, exercise, and sleep on a schedule. Pharmacologic treatments should be governed by a "start low, go slow" philosophy: a mono-sequential approach to prescribing – adding a single agent, titrating until the targeted behavior is reduced, side effects become intolerable, or the maximal dosage is achieved (Rayner et al, 2006). Goals of managing the care of individuals suffering from dementia and the behavioral issues which occur should include symptom reduction and preservation of quality of life.

Stages of Alzheimer's disease (AD)

There are common patterns of symptom progression that occur in many individuals with AD and there are many ways to stage the progression. Staging systems provide useful frames of reference for understanding how the disease may present in individuals. But it is important to note that not everyone will experience the same symptoms of the disease or progress at the same rate. Alzheimer's disease can run its course in 4 years, but some individuals live 20 years with the disease (Alzheimer's Organization, 2010). The following outlines the key symptoms characterizing the four stages if AD, ranging from early to the terminal stage.

Early Stage of Alzheimer's disease (AD)

- Decreased attention span
- Less motivated to complete tasks
- Gets lost in familiar places
- Problems with language – uses substitute words or words that rhyme
- Misplaces things or puts things in strange places
- Trouble with abstract thinking
- Changes in mood & personality – can become depressed or irritable
- Apathetic, withdrawn, avoids people
- Anxious, irritable, agitated
- Insensitive to other's feelings
- Easily angered
- Frustrates easily, tires easily, feels rushed, surprises easily
- Idiosyncratic behaviors start to develop
- Hoards, checks for items repeatedly, or searches for objects of little value
- Forgets to eat or eats constantly

Moderate Stage of AD

- Increasing difficulty in sorting out names & faces of family and friends
- Is able to distinguish familiar from unfamiliar
- Still knows own name
- No longer remembers addresses or phone numbers
- Can no longer think logically or clearly
- Cannot organize own speaking or follow logic of others
- Unable to follow written or oral instructions
- Unable to sequence steps, follow a series of instructions
- Arithmetic & money problems escalate
- Disorientated
- Issues with season, day of week, time of day
- Poor short term memory
- Repeats questions over and over, or tells the same story again and again
- Forgets recent events
- Forgets names and words – may make up stories to fill in their own gaps in memory
- Very poor abstract thinking

Late Stage of AD

- Mental abilities decline
- Personality changes
- Physical problems begin
- Complete deterioration of personality
- Abnormal limb movements
- Cognition declines-the individual is unable to follow a series of instructions or commands as well as unable to carry on a conversation
- Appears uncomfortable
- Can cry when touched or moved
- Can no longer smile
- Either unable to speak or speaks incoherently
- Cannot write or comprehend reading material
- Loses voluntary control of bodily functions
- Urinary and/or bowel incontinence
- Unable to walk, stand, sit up, or hold head up without assistance
- Cannot swallow easily
- Pockets food or medicines in mouths
- Chokes easily
- Cannot move voluntarily

Terminal Stage of AD

- Unable to swallow
- Increased incidence of choking/aspiration
- Becomes contracted in fetal position
- Increased incidence of pressure ulcers
- Incontinent of urine and feces
- Increased incidence of urinary tract infections
- Increased incidence of constipation/fecal impactions
- Decreased respiratory movements
- Increases incidence of respiratory infections & pneumonia
- Immune system fails
- Unable to fight off infection
- Recurrent Urinary Tract infections
- Recurrent Pneumonias
- Death

Confusion and disorientation are common occurrences for individuals who have a diagnosis of dementia. This can make it increasingly difficult for the person to maintain a normal life, due to the behavioral issues presented. Memory impairment and delusional beliefs are common in elders with dementia and may result in inappropriate behaviors in social situations or even at home, resulting in difficult situations. Psychotic behaviors such as hallucinations (usually visual), delusions, and delusional misidentifications can also present in individuals with dementia.

Hallucinations are false sensory perceptions that are not merely distortions or misinterpretations

Delusions are beliefs about events that are untrue, but the events are not out of context with a person's social and cultural background

Delusional misidentification may result from a combined decline in visual function and recent memory problems: individuals may suspect that a family member is an impostor, believe that strangers are living in their home, or fail to recognize their own reflection in a mirror

Other troubling issues can include non-psychotic behaviors associated with dementia: agitation, wandering, sexual disinhibition, and aggression

The goals of treatment for any type of dementia are to slow the decline of cognition, maintain independence, and optimize the quality of life for these individuals.

Delirium or Extreme Anxiety

Delirium is a sudden severe confusion with rapid changes in mentation – occurring over a few hours to a few days with markedly increased changes in level of consciousness, including anxiety and agitation. Delirium usually has a treatable cause and, once treated, the person returns to their baseline of level of consciousness, orientation, and functioning.

Common causes of delirium in elders
- Urinary tract infection (UTI)
- Upper respiratory infection (URI)
- Constipation
- Dehydration
- Hyperthyroidism or Hypothyroidism
- Depression
- Urinary Incontinence
- Urinary Retention
- Endocrine or other neurological problem
- Reduced Sensory input
  o Visual disturbances
  o Deafness
  o Sudden changes in environment
- Medications (over-the-counter, as well as prescription)
  o antidepressants with stimulating properties or caffeine can cause or exacerbate anxiety

Sundowning

'Sundowning' is a behavior that can occur in individuals with dementia. It is an increase in confusion and an increase in the occurrence of problematic behaviors in the late afternoon, early evening, and/or night-time hours, including agitation, aggression, and wandering. Sundowning is most commonly seen in individuals suffering from Alzheimer's disease, but also occurs in individuals suffering from other dementias. Sundowning behaviors can occur as early in the day as 2 to 3 pm, but the most commonly-reported time of occurrence is between 6 and 8 pm (Haggerly, 2002). There are several causes of sundowning, including increased fatigue (which can result in a decreased ability to tolerate stressful situations such as a noisy dinnertime or bedtime routines); or increasing confusion, hallucinations, or delusions at night, due to darkness and shadows. The best way to diminish sundowning behaviors is to establish a routine and engage the person involved in a non-demanding activity during the time the sundowning behaviors usually occur. For example, make late afternoons and evenings as simple and non-demanding as possible. Have the person fold washcloths in the afternoon – a repetitive, constructive activity. It is beneficial to reduce distractions and unscheduled activities at the times when these troubling behaviors usually escalate. Try to schedule routine activities, such as bathing, in the morning when the person is more rested. In the evening, keep rooms well-lit until bedtime to diminish shadows and hallucinations.

Neuropsychological Testing

Neuropsychological testing studies an individual's behavior and mood, and attempts to offer a definitive diagnosis when confusion presents in a person. It is utilized when an individual is having significant problems with memory, concentration, understanding, visual-spatial issues, and a variety of other symptoms. It is useful in differentiating between Alzheimer's disease and other various psychiatric problems, like depression and anxiety, problems caused by medications, issues of substance abuse, strokes, and tumors. Neuropsychological testing is a lengthy process administered over an average of 8 hours; it encompasses a comprehensive interview with the person and may include tests to assess memory, language, the ability to plan and reason, and the ability to modify behavior, as well as assessments of personality and emotional stability (WebMD, 2010).

Mini-Mental State Exam

The Mini-Mental Status Examination (MMSE), developed by Dr. Marshal Folstein and Dr. Susan Folstein, offers a quick and simple way to quantify cognitive function and screen for cognitive loss. It is not a diagnostic test, but a test which can follow the progression of the disease in an individual when the test is administered periodically and that person's scores are compared – to show improvement in cognition, stabilization in cognition, or decline in cognition. It tests the individual's orientation, attention, calculation, recall, language and motor skills and each section involves a series of questions or commands. The individual receives one point for each correct answer. The administrator of the test is seated with an individual in a quiet, well-lit room. The individual is asked to listen carefully and to answer each question as accurately as he/she can. The test is not timed but the scoring is immediate.

An individual can receive a maximum score of 30 points. In general, a score between 25 and 30 indicates adequate cognitive functioning: scores between 24 and 20 indicate mild cognitive impairment, between 19 and 10 usually indicates moderate cognitive impairment, and a score below 10 indicates severe cognitive impairment. The raw score may need to be corrected for educational level and age. Low scores may indicate the presence of dementia, although other mental disorders can also lead to abnormal findings. Physical problems can also interfere with interpretation if not properly noted; for example, an individual is unable to hear or read instructions properly, or may have a motor deficit that affects writing and drawing skills, causing the scores to be abnormally low (Wikipedia, 2010). Despite the many free versions of the test that are available on the internet, the official version is copyrighted and must be ordered through Psychological Assessment Resources (PAR).

Clock Drawing Test

The Clock Drawing Test (CDT) is a simple test that can be used as a part of a neurological test or as a simple screening tool for Alzheimer's and other types of dementia. The test can provide information about general cognitive and adaptive functioning such as memory, processing information, and visual-spatial issues. It is highly correlated with the MMSE and a normal clock drawing almost always correlates with normal cognitive abilities (Kennard, 2006).

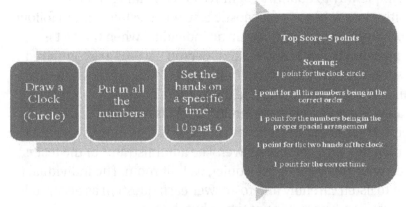

Figure 8-1. *Clock Drawing Test*

Mini-Cog Test

The Mini-Cog is a very simple and quick test which takes about 3 minutes to administer and is often used to assist in identifying people who require further investigation into their clinical situation. The test consists of a three item recall and a clock drawing test. First, a person is asked to remember 3 items and then is asked to draw a clock – the same as the Clock Drawing Test (CDT). Next the person is asked to recall the three words. Scoring: If a person is unable to recall 3 words – he/she has some form of dementia; if able to name 1 to 2 words and able to perform an adequate CDT – he/she probably does not have does not have Alzheimer's dementia; if able to name 1 to 2 words and unable to perform an adequate CDT – he/she is probably has some form of dementia; and if is able to recall all 3 items – he/she probably does not have an Alzheimer's type of dementia, the individual may have another type of dementia or not have dementia but another problem, depending upon other symptoms presented (Kennard, 2006).

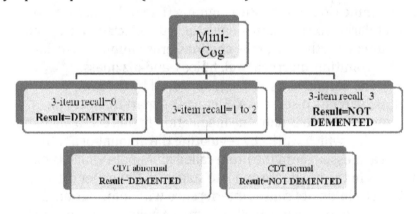

Figure 8-2. *Mini-Cog Test*

Treatment for Alzheimer's disease

Treatment for Alzheimer's disease (AD) consists of slowing the progression of the disease, improving quality of life, and managing the problems caused by the disease. There are several different types of medications used to treat the associated memory loss, behavior changes, sleep problems, and the other symptoms of AD.

There are two classes of drugs that are approved by the Food and Drug Administration (FDA) specifically for treating Alzheimer's disease (AD). The medications aim to manage the chemical imbalances within the brain in order to improve cognition, slow the progression of the disease, and diminish behavioral problems. In the brain of an individual with AD, acetylcholine is destroyed too rapidly, making it difficult for the signals to be transmitted along the neural pathway. Cholinesterase inhibitors are used to slow the destruction and slow the progression of AD as well as help improve cognitive symptoms. These medications work by preventing the breakdown of a chemical messenger in the brain called acetylcholine which is important for learning, memory, and attention. There are three cholinesterase inhibitors approved for the treatment of AD: Donepezil (Aricept) which is indicated and approved to treat mild, moderate, and severe Alzheimer's; Rivastigmine (Exelon) and Galantamine (Razadyne). Rivastigmine (Exelon) is also approved to treat Parkinson's disease dementia. Side effects that have been associated with the use of the cholinesterase inhibitors include nausea, vomiting, diarrhea, weight loss, and dizziness.

The second class of drugs approved by the FDA to treat Alzheimer's disease is N-Methyl D-Aspartate Receptor Antagonists. There is only one medication in this class: Memantine (Namenda), which works by regulating the amount of another chemical messenger in the brain called glutamate which is made in excess in the moderate and late stages of Alzheimer's disease. Excessive glutamate causes interference with information retrieval and memory as well as increase behavioral problems. Namenda is indicated and approved by the FDA for treating the moderate to severe stages of AD and works by binding with the excessive glutamate. Side effects can include dizziness, confusion, headache, constipation, nausea, and agitation. Since memantine works on a different chemical within the brain than a cholinesterase inhibitor, they are often used in combination.

Other Medications

There are other medications commonly used in caring for individuals with a diagnosis of AD that are aimed at managing the behavioral and psychiatric symptoms such as hallucinations, agitation, and sleep problems. However, none of these medications are indicated or approved by the FDA to treat dementia, including AD. But all of these medications are commonly used and can be found in current literature discussing treatment of behavioral problems exhibited by individuals with dementia. The three main classes of medications include: a) Antidepressants, which treat depression; b) Anxiolytics, which treat anxiety and restlessness; and c) Antipsychotic medications, which treat hallucinations, delusions, agitation, and aggression.

Antidepressants

Depression is common in individuals with a diagnosis of Alzheimer's disease or other types of dementia, and often antidepressant medications are used. The class of drugs most commonly prescribed in the elderly population is the Selective Seratonin Reuptake Inhibitor (SSRI) antidepressants because of their therapeutic efficacy and favorable side-effect profile (Salzman, Schneider, & Alexopoulos, 2010). They are highly selective in treating depression symptoms, are well known for their benign interaction and may offer patients an equally effective, and far safer, alternative to conventional treatment with antipsychotic medications (Rosack, 2002). In certain circumstances, antidepressants have been shown to be just as effective as an antipsychotic for calming agitation and treating psychotic symptoms in older individuals with dementia (Pollock, 2007). There are other classes of antidepressant medications, but the SSRIs are the class of choice in the geriatric population.

Anxiolytics

Anxiety is another common problem in individuals with a diagnosis of dementia. Anxiolytics are a class of anti-anxiety medications used to treat anxiety presented by individuals suffering from dementia. They work by calming and relaxing a person and may be prescribed in conjunction with other medications to relieve anxiety symptoms (eHow, 2010). Anxiolytics are good agents to use when a confused individual is unable to be consoled, redirected, or calmed and there is a potential for injury to self or others. They can produce side effects such as sleepiness, fainting, dizziness, blurred vision, confusion and potential falls (due to the effects on an individual's balance). There are risks for use of this class if it is prescribed in high doses. There are potential interactions with alcohol or other drugs, that cause depression of brain functioning which can cause depression in respirations and potentially cause a person to stop breathing. Anxiolytics should be used cautiously, but they may be necessary when an individual is unable to function and has a poor quality of life due to anxiety, paranoia, or extreme delusions.

Antipsychotic Medications

Antipsychotic medications are not indicated for treatment of Alzheimer's disease, but they are commonly used in individuals with a diagnosis of dementia to treat hallucinations, delusions, or extreme 'sundowning' behaviors. Antipsychotic medications are being used to decrease the psychosis or agitated behaviors associated with dementia and to calm the racing thoughts, paranoia, and agitation. This allows a person to interact with other people, follow a routine, and be as independent as possible. This class of medications must not be used as a chemical restraint (which is the use of a medication to quiet a person and make the person sedated). Antipsychotic medications may be used to enhance quality of life for an individual who exhibits distressing and agitated behaviors which endanger the person and/or others. The benefits of using this type of medication must be weighed against the risks associated with its use. It is important to note that there have been medical problems associated with antipsychotic medication use in older individuals. The adverse effects that can be caused by an antipsychotic medication may include an increased risk of strokes and death in individuals suffering from dementia, worsening of diabetes and worsening of cholesterol problems, increases a person's risks for falling; antipsychotic medications currently have a "black box" warning issued by the FDA about their use in older patients with dementia for increased risks of causing death. Antipsychotic medications can cause dystonia, which are abnormal, repetitious, involuntary movements in individuals (such as constant tongue protrusion, constant chewing, rocking motions, pill rolling, etc.). If an individual develops dystonic movements, a medication's use must be re-evaluated to determine if it is in the person's best interest to continue use or if the medication should be discontinued. Appropriate laboratory monitoring is required with the use of all of the antipsychotic medications including: laboratory tests to monitor liver and kidney functioning, Glucose and Hgb A1C to monitor status of diabetes, and cholesterol panels at least every 6 months. Attempts should be made to wean or discontinue the use of an antipsychotic medication if the person is no longer exhibiting distressing behaviors. Weaning an antipsychotic should be done slowly and the individual monitored for problems re-emerging as the medication is decreased.

Additional Medications

There are additional medications used in the management of the symptoms of Alzheimer's disease and other dementias. Anticonvulsants have been used to manage behavioral problems presented in individuals with a diagnosis of dementia. The most commonly used drug in this class is Divalproic Acid (Depakote), which has been used to treat seizures, bipolar disorder and migraine headaches. Psychiatrists observed that Depakote had certain side effects, which included calming of anxious behaviors. It began to be used for these effects on mood and behavior in individuals with behavioral problems. This medication dampens the speed and frequency with which neurons fire. In addition to assisting in managing the symptoms of anxiety, agitation, and psychotic behaviors in individuals with dementia, scientists think that Depakote may also inhibit the development of the plaques and tangle formation in the brains of Alzheimer's patients (Peterson, 2004). This medication should be used cautiously in individuals, because it has the potential to cause sedation, falls, and orthostatic hypotension. There is a "black box" warning for liver damage and use of this medication requires routine monitoring of liver function and drug levels. Be aware that a Depakote drug level in an individual's blood does not need to be in the drug's therapeutic range, since it is not being used to treat seizures in these individuals – drug levels are being done to monitor for and prevent toxicity.

Other Medications commonly used to treat the problems associated with Alzheimer's disease Medications

Other Alzheimer's Therapies

Several non-prescription medication therapies are being used to help Alzheimer's patients cope with the symptoms of the disease.

Sensory therapies There is evidence that sensory therapies such as music therapy and art therapy can improve Alzheimer's patients' mood, behavior, and day-to-day function. By stimulating the senses, these therapies may help trigger memory recall and enable individuals with a diagnosis of Alzheimer's disease to reconnect with the world around them.

Alternative therapies Some people have tried alternative remedies, including coenzyme Q10, coral calcium, huperzine A, and omega-3 fatty acids to prevent or treat Alzheimer's disease. However, there is no proven efficacy of these treatments to suggest recommending the use of any of these agents as an Alzheimer's therapy. And, because these are supplements, the FDA does not regulate them as it does prescription medications. Caution must be used, since all dietary and nutritional supplements have the potential to cause dangerous side effects or interact with other medications an individual may be taking.

Lifestyle changes might help slow cognitive decline in people with Alzheimer's. For example, studies have shown that eating a Mediterranean diet (which is high in fish, nuts, and healthy oils) may reduce the risk of an individual developing Alzheimer's disease, and that exercise may improve the symptoms of the disease as well.

Researchers are looking into several new treatment options for Alzheimer's. One of the most promising Alzheimer's therapies in development focuses on beta amyloid. Researchers are trying to develop new therapies that prevent beta amyloid from forming, or break it down before it leads to Alzheimer's (Web MD, 2010).

Other Dementias Lewy Body, Picks Disease, Parkinson's disease, and Other Neurodegenerative disorders.

A discussion of the various causes of dementia includes the physical as well as psychiatric changes and problems occurring. Current treatment plans to manage these disorders will be discussed including common diagnostic testing and management strategies (behavioral, environmental, and pharmacological)

Dementia is the loss of mental functions, including the ability to think, remember, and reason, that is severe enough to interfere with an individual's daily life. In addition to changes in memory, there can be changes in personality, mood, and behavior. Dementia is not a disease but a group of symptoms that is caused by various diseases or conditions. Although Alzheimer's disease is the most common cause of dementia, there are many other causes of dementia, including vascular disease, Lewy Body disorder, Pick's disease, Parkinson's disease, and other neurological disorders. Some individuals will be suffering from a combination of dementias, since certain dementias have similar risk factors; for example, some individuals will have Alzheimer's disease (AD) in addition to another type of dementia.

Vascular Dementia

Vascular dementia is the second most common cause of dementia behind Alzheimer's disease, accounting for up to 20% of all dementias in the older population (MedicineNet, 2010). It is caused by brain damage caused due to cerebrovascular or cardiovascular disease and can be a result of a stroke or a hemorrhagic bleed within the brain. It often coexists with AD. The risks factors for vascular dementia increase with age and a sedentary lifestyle, as well as other concurrent conditions such as hypertension, hypercholesterolemia, diabetes, and obesity.

Risk Factors for Vascular Dementia

- Increasing age is one of the biggest risk factors for vascular disease and vascular dementia. Vascular dementia is rare before the age of 65. People in their 80s and 90s are much more likely to have this disorder than people in their 60s and 70s.
- History of stroke which causes brain damage appears to increase the risk of developing vascular dementia.
- Atherosclerosis is plaque build-up in the arteries and veins which narrows the blood vessels to the brain and thus impedes blood flow to the tissues. This increases the risks of strokes and brain damage and thus increases the risk of developing vascular dementia.
- High blood pressure or Hypertension puts extra pressure on blood vessels throughout the body including the brain. This increases the risk of vascular problems in the brain.
- Diabetes can leads to elevated glucose levels, which can cause damage to blood vessels throughout the body and increase the risk for strokes and other vascular problems in the brain.
- Smoking increases the risk of atherosclerosis and vascular diseases, as well as vascular dementia.
- High cholesterol (which is elevated levels of cholesterol) increases the risk of developing vascular disease, especially in individuals who have high LDL (the bad cholesterol). These individuals are at an increased risk of developing Alzheimer's disease.

(Mayo Clinic-Vascular Dementia, 2010)

Types of Vascular Dementia

Vascular dementia can have a gradual onset over a long period of time or it can begin suddenly, frequently occurring after a sudden event such as a stroke. The symptoms may or may not worsen with time or the symptoms could improve with time. When the symptoms do worsen, they can progress in a stepwise manner, showing gradual decline over time, or with sudden changes in a person's physical functioning or cognitive abilities. Unlike individuals with AD, people with vascular dementia often do not have personality changes, except for depressive symptoms. Emotional responsiveness generally remains normal until the later stages of this type of dementia (MedicineNet, 2010).

There are several types of vascular dementia, including multi-infarct dementia (MID) (which is caused by numerous small strokes in the brain) and Binswanger's disease (a rare form of dementia which is caused by a gradual diminishing of blood flow to the brain). MID typically affects multiple areas of the brain. The cause of damage to the brain in vascular dementia is the impediment of the blood supply to brain tissue caused by an occlusion – a stroke – or caused by a hemorrhagic bleed within the brain. Essentially, the damage to the brain occurs due to either a lack of blood flow or small clots blocking blood flow resulting in brain damage, called infarcts. Binswager's disease is characterized by widespread damage to the brain with injury to multiple small blood vessels that lead to increased atrophy within the brain. There can also be extensive lesions in the white matter or nerve fibers of the brain. Binswanger's disease leads to brain lesions, loss of memory, disordered thinking, and behavior as well as mood changes. Individuals with Binswanger's disease often show signs of abnormal blood pressure, stroke, blood abnormalities, disease of the large blood vessels in the neck, and/or disease of the heart valves (MedicineNet, 2010). Other prominent features include urinary incontinence, difficulty with the ability to walk, clumsiness, slowness, lack of facial expression, and speech difficulty. Treatment of Binswanger's disease is symptomatic and may include the use of medications to manage hypertension, depression, heart arrhythmias, and hypotension (low blood pressure). There may be improvement of symptoms with episodes of partial recovery.

Symptoms of Vascular Dementia

The symptoms of vascular dementia can vary from one individual to another, depending on the portion of the brain that is affected. Adding to the confusion, Alzheimer's disease and vascular dementia frequently occur together. In fact, some believe that having both problems is more common than just having one disorder – Vascular dementia or Alzheimer's dementia (Mayo Clinic, 2010).

Individuals with vascular dementia often experience:

- Confusion
- Agitation
- Memory impairment
- Unsteady gait
- Urinary frequency, urgency or incontinence
- Night wandering
- Depression
- Decline in organizational thinking
- Difficulty planning ahead
- Trouble communicating details sequentially
- Memory loss
- Poor attention
- Poor concentration

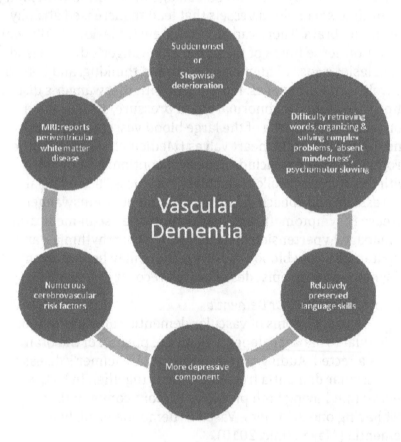

Figure 8-3. *Vascular Dementia*

Diagnosing Vascular Dementia

Diagnosing vascular dementia begins with a full medical work-up, including a physical examination and laboratory tests. Radiological tests may be ordered to explore the possibility of strokes, cerebral hemorrhage, and brain tumors.

Testing for Vascular Dementia

The following tests are often performed to rule out other conditions in individuals with memory impairment or individuals who are confused. One or more tests may be done in order to determine the cause of confusion. If a person is extremely confused, the individual may not be able to cooperate in order to have some of these tests conducted. A test's benefits must be weighed against the risks of conducting a test. For example, if a person must be sedated to have the test done or if the person risks injury to self when having the test performed, then a test may be more burdensome than beneficial and the test omitted. Sometimes it is beneficial to conduct psychiatric testing in addition to tests or in place of a test.

Computerized tomography (CT) (also referred to as a CAT scan or CT scan) uses X-ray equipment to produce a cross-sectional image showing sections of a person's brain. Sometimes a contrast material may be injected to help highlight any abnormalities in the brain's blood vessels.

Magnetic resonance imaging (MRI) uses radio waves and a strong magnetic field to produce detailed images of the brain. In some cases, contrast material may be injected to produce even more detailed pictures. Advances in MRI imaging, as well as expertise in interpreting these results, have resulted in the MRI becoming an excellent tool for distinguishing between vascular dementia, Alzheimer's disease, and other dementias.

Positron emission tomography (PET) is a scan of the brain after a person is injected with a low-level radioactive material that binds to chemicals which travel to a person's brain. This helps show which parts of the brain are not functioning properly. The test is painless and can be particularly useful in distinguishing between different types of dementia.

Doppler ultrasound uses high-frequency sound waves to measure the direction and speed of blood cells as they travel through blood vessels known as carotid arteries, which supply blood to a person's brain. A Doppler ultrasound of a person's carotid arteries can help detect blockages or narrowing vessels that impede blood flow to the brain.

Neuropsychological testing assesses orientation, learning, recall, attention, calculation and language. Individuals with vascular dementia typically exhibit the same types of cognitive deficits as individuals with Alzheimer's disease. One major difference, however, is in memory function. Most individuals with vascular dementia do not experience short-term memory problems until later in the course of the disease, unless there is a stroke in the exact area of the brain that controls memory. (Mayo Clinic, 2010)

Treating Vascular Dementia

There is no cure for vascular dementia and no drugs have been approved by the Food and Drug Administration (FDA) to treat this problem. Most medications that are used are designed to treat the symptoms of Alzheimer's disease, which often appears concurrently with vascular dementia. These medications have been shown to help improve confusion, as well as treat mood and behavioral problems in individuals with vascular dementia.

Cholinesterase inhibitors – donepazil (Aricept), galantamine (Razadyne) and rivastigmine (Exelon) – are approved as treatment for Alzheimer's disease and work by slowing the destruction of acetylcholine, a chemical messenger that plays a key role in memory and judgment. These medications are sometimes used in individuals with vascular dementia since Alzheimer's disease and vascular disease often co-exist in elders.

N-Methyl-D-Aspartate Receptor Antagonist (NMDA) – Memantine (Namenda) has been shown to provide a modest benefit in individuals who have vascular dementia. Memantine works by regulating glutamate, a chemical messenger involved in information processing, storage and retrieval.

Antidepressants/Mood stabilizers – Selective Serotonin Reuptake Inhibitors (SSRI) are antidepressants that may be just as effective as an antipsychotic for calming agitation and treating psychotic symptoms in older individuals with vascular dementia (Pollock, 2007).

Valproate (Divalproic Acid or Depakote) – is indicated to treat seizure disorders, but also has an anti-aggressivity property that has demonstrated an ability to augment brain GABA and serotonin concentrations, thereby helping in the management of agitation/aggression in individuals with dementia (Guay & Lott, 2010).

Other Medications – Efforts are also aimed at managing the risk factors for developing vascular dementia, including managing hypertension, lowering cholesterol levels, controlling diabetes, and possibly thinning an individual's blood with use of aspirin or an anti-platelet aggregator medication, such as ticlopidine (Ticlid) and clopidogrel (Plavix). This is to help prevent blood clots. Certain individuals may also be taking a blood thinner known as warfarin (Coumadin). None of these measures can reverse the problems caused by vascular dementia, so most efforts are aimed at preventing further damage (Mayo Clinic, 2010).

Lewy Body Dementia

Lewy body dementia shares similar characteristics of both Alzheimer's disease (AD) and Parkinson's disease dementia (PDD). Like AD, it causes confusion. Like PDD, it can result in rigid muscles, slowed movement and tremors. Individuals with Lewy Body dementia (LBD) have abnormal microscopic protein deposits within the mid-brain called 'Lewy Bodies'.

These deposits, which have been found in nerve cells, can cause disruption to the brain's normal functioning, causing it to slowly deteriorate. They were first discovered in 1912 by Frederick Lewy; this is where the name of the disorder was derived (HelpGuide, 2010).

The most striking symptoms of LBD are hallucinations, which can be one of the first signs of this disorder. Hallucinations may include visual hallucinations (ranging from seeing abstract shapes or colors to visions of animals and people) or auditory hallucinations (hearing sounds or voices that are not real). There can be instances where the individual with LBD has conversations with a visual hallucination – for example, the person with LBD has a conversation with a deceased loved one. LBD is estimated to affect less than 1 percent of the population over the age of 65 (Crystal, 2009).

Risk Factors for Lewy Body Dementia (LBD)
LBD has several factors that appear to increase an individual's risk of developing the disease:

Advanced Age – Most cases of LBD occur in individuals over the age of 60.

Gender – LBD is more common in men.

Heredity – LBD appears to have a genetic link; if a person has a family member who has LBD, the risks for developing the disease are increased.

Diagnosing LBD
The criteria for a diagnosis of LBD are based on a progressive decline in the ability the person to think, as well as two of the following:
- Fluctuating alertness and cognition, but generally good short-term memory
- Visual hallucinations
- Auditory hallucinations
- Parkinson's-like symptoms, including tremors and pill-rolling motions, slow & rigid movements, and muscle stiffness
- Repeated falls due to the Parkinson-like gait

o Walking with short & shuffling steps, arms at sides and not swinging one's arms with walking, stooped posture with head looking down at feet, and shoulders hunched forward, which throws off a person's center of balance
* Sleep disturbances, including insomnia and the person acting out dreams
* Delusions or depression
* Fluctuations in autonomic processes, including blood pressure, body temperature, urinary difficulties, constipation, and difficulty swallowing
* Day-to-day symptom variability

LBD Testing

No single test can diagnose LBD; the diagnosis is made through the process of a medical work-up and eliminating or ruling out other diseases and conditions that may cause similar signs and symptoms. Tests may include:

Neurological exam should be part of the physical exam, assessing for signs of Parkinson's disease, strokes, tumors or other medical conditions that can impair brain function, as well as physical function.

Mental status exam assesses an individual's memory and thinking abilities. Initially, an abbreviated version should be done and, if warranted, a longer version with neuropsychological testing should administered by trained professionals. This can help distinguish normal aging changes from abnormal ones and may help identify patterns in cognitive functions that provide clues to the underlying condition.

Electroencephalogram (EEG) If confusion comes and goes, an EEG may be recommended to help determine if the symptoms are caused by seizures or Creutzfeldt-Jakob disease, a very rare degenerative brain disorder more commonly known as 'mad-cow' disease. This is a painless test which records the electrical activity in an individual's brain.

Brain scans – An MRI or CT scan can examine for evidence of stroke or bleeding and will rule out the possibility of a tumor. (Mayo Clinic, 2010)

Treating LBD

Individuals with LBD are often difficult to manage, due to the behavioral problems which they manifest. There is no cure for LBD; there are not even treatments which can slow the disease. Treatments are aimed at managing the symptoms, setting limits, and constructing a safe and structured environment.

Medications for LBD

Cholinesterase inhibitors – Alzheimer's medications work by increasing the levels of acetylcholine, a neurotransmitter or chemical messenger in the brain believed to be important for memory, thought and judgment. They can help improve alertness, improve cognition, and may help reduce hallucinations and other behavioral problems. The benefits are often small and sometimes not even noticeable

Parkinson's disease medications can help reduce Parkinson's-like muscular symptoms in some individuals with LBD, but can also cause increased confusion, hallucinations and delusions.

Other Medications may help control behavior problems caused by a loss of judgment, increased impulsivity, and confusion. Possible medications include:

Mood stabilizers – Selective Serotonin Reuptake Inhibitors (SSRI) are antidepressants which may be just as effective as an antipsychotic for calming agitation and treating psychotic symptoms in older individuals with dementia (Pollock, 2007).

Valproate (Divalproic Acid or Depakote) – A medication indicated to treat seizure disorders which also has an anti-aggressivity property and an ability to augment an individual's brain GABA and serotonin concentrations. Valproate has been shown to be efficacious in the management of agitation/aggression in individuals with dementia (Guay & Lott, 2010).

Stimulants (such as methylphenidate) are not commonly used, but have been shown to be of some benefit in the management of explosive behavior in adults who have not outgrown their hyperactivity. They are also used to treat certain individuals who exhibit autistic-like behaviors with coexisting hyperactivity and aggression. However, in some individuals, these agents may actually worsen aggressiveness and self-injurious behavior (Guay & Lott, 2010).

Antipsychotic medications are indicated to treat bipolar disorder and psychosis. They have been used to manage behavioral problems in certain individuals. They have been shown to help improve delusions and hallucinations – BUT at least a third of the people who have LBD have a dangerous sensitivity to this class of medications. Reactions can be severe enough to be life-threatening or can be pronounced as seizure-like activity, severe psychosis, or worsening of confusion and agitation (haloperidol, risperdal, olanzapine). They should not be used to treat individuals with Lewy Body dementia.

Parkinson agents – Levodopa is often used to treat the Parkinson-like motor symptoms, but may increase the hallucinations and aggravate other symptoms, such as agitation and delusions.

Managing Behaviors associating with LBD:

All Therapies must include Environmental Structuring

      Since antipsychotic medications can worsen the symptoms of LBD, limit setting and a stable environment are paramount in keeping the individual with LBD and others, safe:

Modify the environment. Reducing clutter and distracting noise can make it easier for someone with LBD to focus and function.

Modify the response. A caregiver's response to a behavior can make the behavior worse. To avoid increasing agitation, the caregiver should not to correct or quiz a person with LBD unless the person's actions are dangerous to self or others. Reassuring the person and validating his or her concerns can defuse most situations.

Modify tasks. Break tasks into easier steps and focus on success, not failure. Structure and routine also help people with LBD feel safe.

Parkinson disease dementia (PDD)

Parkinson's disease is a progressive disorder of the central nervous system which causes slowness of movements, compromise of balance, muscle rigidity, and tremors. The disease is caused by low levels of a chemical called dopamine, which activates the cells in a person's brain that make a person's muscles move. Individuals who develop Parkinson's disease earlier than 40 years of age usually do not develop dementia until late in life, usually after 70 years of age. But individuals who develop the physical symptoms of Parkinson's disease late in life – usually after the age of 60, tend to develop dementia relatively rapidly, usually within 5 years after onset of the disease. The key features associated with PDD are cognitive impairment, including slowing in the ability to think, reduced attention span, and impairment in executive function, such as planning, organizing, and solving problems. An individual may become obsessional, experience loss of emotional control, and exhibit outbursts of anger. Certain medications may cause or aggravate delusions (false beliefs) as well as visual hallucinations. The person may experience language problems, such as stuttering and slower speech, but will not have difficulty finding the correct word (Mayo Clinic, 2010).

Risk factors for developing Parkinson's disease

Age – Middle-aged adults who develop Parkinson's disease very rarely experience the dementia associated with Parkinson's disease until very late in late in life (>70). Parkinson's disease ordinarily begins in middle or late life, and the risk of developing dementia associated with the disease increases if an individual develops Parkinson's disease after the age of 60. The progression of the disease is usually rapid over 2-10 years.

Heredity – There appears to be a genetic link and having one or more close relatives with Parkinson's disease increases a person's chances of developing the disease, although one's risk is still less than 5 percent.

Gender – Men are more likely to develop Parkinson's disease than women.

Exposure to toxins – There has been an association with ongoing exposure to herbicides and pesticides which places a person at a slightly increased risk of developing Parkinson's disease dementia. (Mayo Clinic, 2010)

Symptoms of Parkinson's disease

Most of the symptoms of Parkinson's disease involve disruption of motor functions. Other symptoms include lack of energy, mood and memory changes, and pain.

Primary symptoms of Parkinson's disease

Bradykinesia – slowness in voluntary movement, such as standing up, walking, and sitting down, due to a delay in transmission of signals from the brain to the muscles, which may lead to difficulty initiating movement. But this problem can also lead to more severe problems such as "freezing episodes" (when a person is unable to move and stops once walking has been initiated)

Tremors often occur in the hands, fingers, forearms, foot, mouth, or chin; typically, the tremors take place when the limbs are at rest as opposed to when there is movement

Rigidity or stiff muscle tone often produces muscle pain that is increased during movement

Poor balance – due to the loss of reflexes that help posture, causing unsteady balance, which often leads to falls

Secondary symptoms of Parkinson's disease

- Constipation
- Difficulty swallowing
- Choking, coughing, or drooling
- Excessive salivation
- Excessive sweating
- Loss of bowel and/or bladder control
- Loss of intellectual capacity
- Anxiety, depression, isolation
- Scaling, dry skin on the face or scalp
- Slow response to questions
- Small cramped handwriting
- Soft, whispery voice

(HelpGuide, 2010)

Treatment of Parkinson's disease
There is no cure for Parkinson's disease, but there are several medications used to treat the symptoms of the disease.

Levodopa/Carbidopa (Sinemet) – This is a combination of Levodopa (the chemical that patients with Parkinson's disease lack) and Carbidopa (a chemical that helps the levodopa reach the brain). Its effectiveness tends to decrease after several years and adjustments in dosing may be necessary.

Entacapone (Comtan) is a medication which helps Sinemet work better when it starts to lose its effectiveness. It is also available together with levodopa and carbidopa in a combined product called Stalevo.

Dopamine agonists [ropinorole (Requip) and pramipaxole (Mirapex)] enhance an individual's natural production of dopamine by stimulating the brain. These medications do not have as much risk of long-term side effects as levodopa and they have less chance of losing effectiveness over time in comparison to levodopa. However, there are potential side effects which include dizziness and hallucinations, especially in the elderly or in patients with dementia.

Monoamine oxidase inhibitors [selegiline (Eldepryl and Zelapar) and rasagaline (Azilect)] increase the amount of dopamine available in the brains of individuals with Parkinson's disease. They can be very helpful in a small subset of patients with Parkinson's disease and often have fewer side effects than the dopamine agonists but, they can be harmful when used together with certain other medications, especially some types of antidepressants. Patients can also develop critically elevated blood pressure when taking these medications and eating certain types of foods. (HelpGuide, 2010)

Symptoms of PDD
Dementia is a less common feature of Parkinson's disease; only 20% of individuals with Parkinson's disease develop Parkinson's disease Dementia (PDD). Parkinson's patients who experience hallucinations and more severe motor

control problems are at risk for dementia. For those patients with Parkinson's disease who go on to develop dementia, there is usually at least a 10- to 15-year lag time between their Parkinson's disease diagnosis and the onset of dementia (HelpGuide, 2010). For elders who develop Parkinson's disease after the age of 60, the onset of dementia is more rapid with 20% of these individuals developing dementia within 2 years after the onset of the disease and 50% within 5 years.

Cognitive symptoms in PDD include the following:

- Slowed thinking
- Loss of decision-making ability
- Inflexibility in adapting to changes
- Disorientation in familiar surroundings
- Problems learning new material
- Difficulty concentrating
- Loss of short-term memory progressing to loss of long-term memory
- Difficulty putting a sequence of events in the correct order
- Problems using complex language and comprehending others' complex language

Depression – Sadness, tearfulness, lethargy, withdrawal, loss of interest in activities once enjoyed, insomnia or sleeping too much, weight gain or loss

Anxiety – Excessive worry or fear that disrupts everyday activities or relationships; physical signs, such as restlessness or extreme fatigue, muscle tension, sleeping problems

Psychosis – Inability to think realistically; symptoms can include hallucinations, delusions (false beliefs not shared by others), paranoia (suspicious and feeling controlled by others), and problems thinking clearly; if severe, behavior seriously disrupted; if milder, behavior bizarre, strange, or suspicious

Affect – Mask-like facial expressions

Speech – Slowing, generally hypophonic, some dysarthria and/or stuttering

Testing for PDD

There are no definitive tests that can confirm cognitive decline or dementia in Parkinson's disease. The most accurate way to measure cognitive decline is through conducting neuropsychological testing (eMedicine, 2010). Imaging studies, which include brain scans such as Computerized Tomography (CT) scan and Magnetic Resonance Imaging (MRI), are of little use in diagnosing dementia in individuals with PDD. Positron-emission tomographic (PET) scan may help distinguish dementia from depression and similar conditions.

Treating Parkinson's disease Dementia (PDD)

Cholinesterase inhibitors, specifically Ravistigmine (Exelon) is indicated to treat mild to moderate PDD. They are used to manage the cognitive decline (such as the ability to think and remember), functional decline (such as activities of daily living, including bathing, grooming and toileting), and behavioral problems (such as agitation and argumentative behaviors) (Drugs.com, 2010).

Antidepressants are aimed at treating mood disorders, as well as agitation associated with PDD, and can include tricyclic agents, specifically the secondary amines (e.g., nortriptyline, desipramine), heterocyclic agents, or serotonin reuptake inhibitors (SSRIs), with the SSRIs being the most efficacious and safest in elders.

Anxiolytics - Benzodiazepines may help treat severe anxiety, but side effects such as cognitive impairment and balance problems may be an adverse problem associated with their use. It is paramount that behavior modification techniques are used in conjunction with these medications in the treatment of anxiety. Buspirone is another alternative that is well tolerated, but has not been studied in this population.

Antipsychotic medications are used to treat bipolar disorder and psychosis. They have been used to manage behavioral problems in certain individuals. Clozapine is an older antipsychotic that has been used, but it is no longer commonly used due to the high incidence of adverse effects associated with it. If an antipsychotic is absolutely necessary – Quetiapine (Seroquel) is the antipsychotic of choice in PDD, because it has been shown to help with the cognitive decline, as well as assist in management of psychotic symptoms (Medscape, 2001). Olanzapine and risperidone are also used, but they can worsen motor function and tremors.

Sleep disturbances - Benzodiazepines can be helpful in the treatment of insomnia, as well as rapid eye movement sleep behavior disorder.

(Swanberg & Kalapatapu, 2010)

Pick's disease/Frontotemporal dementia

Pick's disease, or Frontotemporal dementia, refers to a group of dementias that result from hereditary disorders, as well as those that occur spontaneously; e.g., occurring for unknown reasons. This disorder causes the frontal lobe of the brain, and sometimes the temporal lobe of the brain, to degenerate. In this type of dementia, an individual's personality, behavior, and language function are affected more than in Alzheimer's disease. And the person's short-term memory is less affected in Pick's disease (Merck, 2010). Diagnosis is based on symptoms and results of a neurologic examination, as well as the use imaging tests to assess the brain damage. Typically, Pick's disease develops in individuals younger than 65. Men and women are affected equally and this disorder tends to have a heredity component – the incidence of occurrence of Pick's disease increases in individuals with one or more relatives with the disorder. These individuals have abnormal amounts or types of a protein called tau within their brains. In Pick's dementia, the frontal and temporal lobes shrink or atrophy and nerve cells are lost. The affected areas of the brain are generally associated with personality and behavior (Merck, 2010).

Risk Factors for Pick's disease
The only risk factor for Pick's disease is family history; no other risk factors have been found.

Symptoms of Pick's disease
Pick's disease (Frontotemporal dementia) is progressive, but how quickly an individual progresses to general dementia varies. Symptoms include inappropriate behavior, apathy, memory loss, carelessness, and poor personal hygiene. Pick's disease progression varies in each individual – in some, the disease advances to the final stages in less than 2 years; in others, this progression can take up to 10 years.

The 5 Distinguishing Characteristics of Pick's Disease
- Onset before age 65
- Initial personality changes
- Loss of normal controls, such as gluttony, hypersexuality
- Lack of inhibition
- Roaming behavior

(HelpGuide-Pick's disease, 2010)

Symptoms of Pick's disease or Frontotemporal dementia
- Difficulty thinking abstractly
- Difficulty paying attention
- Poor recall
- Remains aware of time, date, and place
- Able to perform daily tasks
- Poor personal hygiene and personal neglect

Changes in Personality and Behavior:
- Some people become uninhibited, resulting in increasingly inappropriate behavior:
  o lacks the ability to follow social rules
    - speaks rudely
    - reacts impulsively
    - abnormal increase in interest in sex
- Impulsivity and compulsiveness
- Repetitious actions
- Wandering or walking in the same location repeatedly
- May compulsively pick up objects or manipulate random objects
- May have an oral fixation and put objects in their mouth, may suck or smack their lips, or may overeat or eat only one type of food

Problems with Language:
- Difficulty finding words
- Difficulty using and/or understanding language (aphasia)
- Dyarthria – physically producing speech becomes more difficult
- Receptive aphasia – Some individuals cannot understand language, but speak fluently, although what the person says does not make any sense
- Anomia – Some have difficulty naming objects
- Prosopagnosia – Some have difficulty recognizing faces
- Speech changes
  - May speak less and less
  - May repeat what they or others say (echolalia)
  - Eventually, they stop speaking

Physical Changes
- In some people, muscles are affected and the individual becomes weak and develops a wasting syndrome (muscles atrophy)
- Muscles of the head and neck are affected – making swallowing, chewing, and talking difficult

(Merck, 2010)

Diagnosing Pick's disease
The diagnosis of Pick's disease (Frontotemporal dementia) is based on symptoms, including how the symptoms develop. Observers may be helpful in diagnosing the disorder because the individuals who are suffering from Pick's disease may be unaware of their symptoms. A neurologic examination and neuropsychiatric testing may be conducted, as well as radiological testing.

Computed tomography (CT) and magnetic resonance imaging (MRI) are done to determine which parts of the brain and how much of the brain is affected. This test can also be done to exclude other possible causes, such as brain tumors, abscesses, or a stroke. However, CT or MRI may not detect the characteristic changes of frontotemporal dementia until late in the disorder.

Positron emission tomography (PET) may help differentiate Pick's disease from other dementias, but often PET is used only in research.

Treatment for Pick's disease
There is no specific treatment for Pick's disease. Generally, treatment is focused upon managing symptoms and providing general support. Speech therapy may help those individuals with language problems.

Antidepressants/Mood stabilizers – Selective Serotonin Reuptake Inhibitors (SSRI) are antidepressants that may assist in calming agitation, decreasing impulsiveness, and treating psychotic symptoms in older individuals with Pick's disease dementia (Pollock, 2007).

Valproate (Divalproate Acid or Depakote) is indicated to treat seizure disorder, but has been used in the management of agitation/aggression in individuals with dementia (Guay & Lott, 2010).

Stimulants (such as methylphenidate) are not commonly used, but have been shown to be of some benefit in the management of impulsive behaviors in individuals who have not outgrown a hyperactive disorder. They are also used to treat individuals with autistic characteristics who have coexisting hyperactivity and aggression. However, in some individuals, these agents may actually worsen aggressiveness and self-injurious behavior (Guay & Lott, 2010).

Antipsychotic medications are indicated to treat bipolar disorder and psychotic behaviors, but may help improve delusions and hallucinations, as well as calm agitated behaviors in individuals with Pick's disease (Pollock, 2007).

Other Dementias

Creutzfeldt-Jakob Disease - This rare disease, which causes a rapidly progressive dementia, can lead to a person's death within a year. The most common early symptoms for this disorder include memory loss and confusion. This disorder may resemble symptoms of other dementias. A variant form of Creutzfeldt-Jakob disease is thought to be acquired from eating beef contaminated with prions. This variant form of this disease causes a dementia similar to that of Creutzfeldt-Jakob disease, except the first symptoms tend to be psychiatric symptoms (such as anxiety or depression), rather than memory loss. There is no current treatment available.

HIV-Associated Dementia - In the late stages of human immunodeficiency virus (HIV) infection, the virus may infect the brain directly and cause damage to nerve cells, resulting in dementia. Dementia may also result from other infections to which people with HIV infection are prone. Unlike almost all other forms of dementia, it tends to occur in younger individuals. This dementia may begin subtly, but progresses steadily over a few months or years and usually occurs after other symptoms of HIV infection are evidenced. Symptoms of this dementia include slowed thinking and expression, difficulty concentrating, and apathy. Abstract thinking and insight are generally not affected. Movements can be slow, muscles weak, and coordination impaired. When HIV infection is diagnosed or when mental function changes in people with HIV infection, computed tomography (CT) or magnetic resonance imaging (MRI) may be done to check for a brain infection or tumors. When confusion occurs in these individuals, a spinal tap, also referred to as lumbar puncture, may be performed to obtain a sample of cerebrospinal fluid for analysis and check for infection, unless evidence suggests that pressure within the skull is increased. An individual's HIV infection may be treated with zidovudine and other drugs, which sometimes produces dramatic improvement. However, because the infection is not cured, dementia may recur (Merck, 2010).

Dementia Pugilistica - A disorder which is also called chronic progressive traumatic encephalopathy and may develop in individuals who have repeated head injuries such as boxers, football players, etc. These individuals often develop symptoms similar to those of Parkinson's disease (e.g., tremors, muscle rigidity, etc), and some of them also develop normal-pressure hydrocephalus.

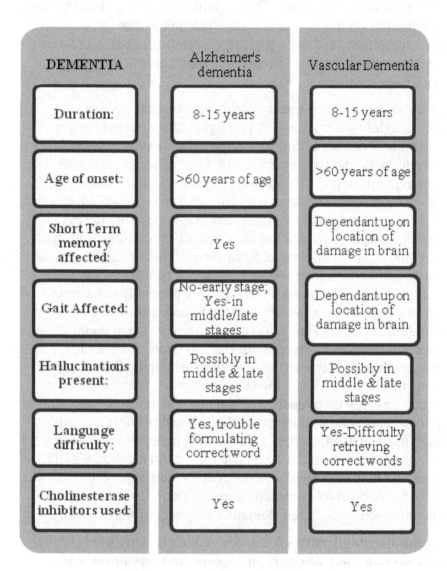

DEMENTIA	Alzheimer's dementia	Vascular Dementia
Duration:	8-15 years	8-15 years
Age of onset:	>60 years of age	>60 years of age
Short Term memory affected:	Yes	Dependant upon location of damage in brain
Gait Affected:	No-early stage; Yes-in middle/late stages	Dependant upon location of damage in brain
Hallucinations present:	Possibly in middle & late stages	Possibly in middle & late stages
Language difficulty:	Yes, trouble formulating correct word	Yes-Difficulty retrieving correct words
Cholinesterase inhibitors used:	Yes	Yes

Figure 8-4. *Comparing the Different Dementias*

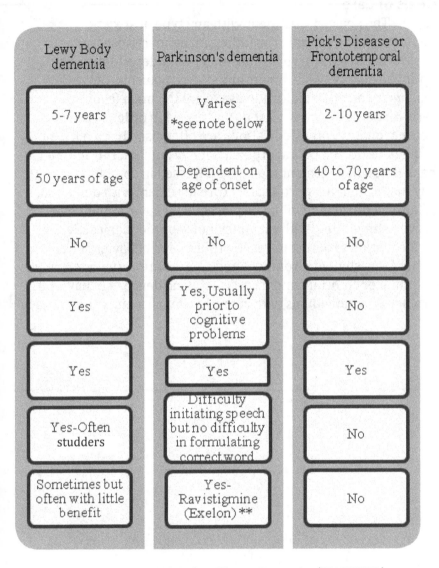

Lewy Body dementia	Parkinson's dementia	Pick's Disease or Frontotemporal dementia
5-7 years	Varies *see note below	2-10 years
50 years of age	Dependent on age of onset	40 to 70 years of age
No	No	No
Yes	Yes, Usually prior to cognitive problems	No
Yes	Yes	Yes
Yes-Often studders	Difficulty initiating speech but no difficulty in formulating correct word	No
Sometimes but often with little benefit	Yes-Rav istigmine (Exelon) **	No

Figure 8-4. *Comparing the Different Dementias (CONTINUED)*

*In individuals with Parkinson's disease dementia, the onset is dependent upon the age of onset of Parkinson's disease: those who develop Parkinson's disease <40 have a later onset of dementia; iIndividuals who develop Parkinson's disease > 60 have a more rapid onset of dementia. (Hitti, 2006)

Goals of Care

The goals of treatment with any type of anxiety, depression, or dementia (including Alzheimer's disease) are to slow the decline of cognition, maintain independence, and optimize quality of life. Environmental structuring, behavioral management, and medication usage are the main focus of care. All of these issues must be addressed in order to provide optimal quality care. Medications are often used but a pill is not a 'quick fix' to behavioral problems. Environment, routine, and behavioral management must be addressed in combination with any medication to appropriately care for elders with dementia. When a confused individual is placed in an environment that is over-stimulating, with too much noise or too many activities or the person's routine is upset, problematic behaviors often occur. Consistent environment and routine are very important to maintain equilibrium and decrease the incidence of behavioral problems in individuals with cognitive impairment or dementia.

Table 8-3. *Medications used in Dementia Care*		

Many of the following medications are not indicated or approved by Food and Drug Administration (FDA) to treat Alzheimer's disease or Dementia.

Medication	Geriatric Dosage Suggestions	Potential Side Effects of Medication
Cholinesterase Inhibitors *indicated for treatment of the early, middle, & late stages of Alzheimer's disease; Rivastigmine is also indicated by the FDA to treat Parkinson's disease dementia*		
donepezil (Aricept)	5 mg daily for 30 days 10 mg daily *New 23 mg daily dose may be used in certain individuals after the person has been on Aricept 10 mg daily for a minimum of 3 months	Most common problems are related to loss of appetite, nausea, vomiting, abdominal pain, and diarrhea
rivastigmine (Exelon)	start at 1.5 mg twice a day for 2 weeks, then 3 mg twice a day for 2 weeks, then 4.5 mg then 6 mg twice a day (max dose-12 mg/day); *Patch is available = 4.6 mg/24 hour – change once a day; after 4 weeks increase to 9.5mg/24 hours	
galantamine (Razadyne)	4 mg twice a day, increase every 4 weeks until reaching12 mg twice a day	
N-Methyl D-Aspartate Receptor Antagonists *indicated by the FDA for treating the middle and late stages of Alzheimer's disease*		
memantine (Namenda)	Titration: Start at 5 mg daily for 7 days, then 5 mg twice a day for 7 days, then 5mg in morning, 10mg in evening for 7 days, then 10 mg twice a day	*Sedation, constipation, dizziness, headache, and pain

(CONTINUED)

Antidepressants – Selective Serotonin Reuptake Inhibitors (SSRI)
indicated by the FDA to treat depression

bupropion (Wellbutrin)	75-100 mg once a day or twice a day	**Entire Class of SSRI: Weight gain, dizziness, somnolence, insomnia, decreased libido, tremors, akathesia, tremors, nervousness, sweating, and various gastrointestinal, as well as sexual, disturbances
duloxetine (Cymbalta)	20-60 mg once a day	
escitalopram (Lexapro)	5-20 mg once a day	
fluoxetine (Prozac)	10-20 mg once a day	
paroxetine (Paxil)	10-40 mg once a day	
paroxetine CR (Paxil CR)	12.5-37.5 mg once a day	
sertraline (Zoloft)	25-50 mg once a day	
venlafaxine XR (Effexor XR)	37.5-150 mg once a day	

Anxiolytics *indicated by the FDA for treatment of anxiety symptoms –*
Not recommended to be used routinely

alprazolam (Xanax)	0.25-0.5 mg every 6 to 8 hours as needed	Sedation, falls, orthostatic hypotension, & increased confusion
clonazepam (Klonipin)	0.125-2 mg every 12 hours as needed (*has a long half-life)	
clorazepate (Tranxene)	3.75-15 mg every 8 hours as needed	
lorazepam (Ativan)	0.5-2mg every 6 to 8 hours as needed (*has the shortest half-life & is the drug of choice, if necessary, in elders with dementia)	

(CONTINUED)

Table 8-3. Medications used in Dementia Care (CONTINUED)

**Antipsychotic medications** *not indicated by the FDA for treating behavioral problems in elders with dementia; indicated for use with agitation and psychosis in individuals with psychosis, bipolar disorder and other psychiatric conditions		
aripiprazole (Abilify)	2-30 mg once or twice a day	Hypotension, seizures, hyperglycemia, worsening of diabetes, weight gain, headache, cataract formation, worsening of depression, & hyperprolactinemia
olanzapine (Zyprexa)	1.25-10 mg once a day at bedtime or twice a day maximum daily dose is 15 mg per day	
quetiapine (Seroquel)	12.5-200 mg once, twice or three times a day	*Antipsychotics have the potential to cause sedation, somnolence or insomnia, orthostatic hypotension, falls, strokes, diabetes, extrapyramidal symptoms, dystonic movements, myocardial infarction, and death
risperidone (Risperdal)	0.25 to 1 mg once or twice a day	
ziprasidone (Geodon)	20-80 mg once or twice a day * QT prolongation, rash, hypertension *must monitor EKGs	
		**all patients receiving drugs in this class must have routine monitoring of liver & kidney functioning, Hgb A1C, Cholesterol

**all patients receiving drugs in this class must have routine monitoring of liver & kidney functioning, Hgb A1C, Cholesterol

**Seizure medication (used for its side effect of calming behavioral problems)** *indicated by the FDA for treatment of seizure disorder and not indicated by the FDA for use of managing behavioral problems in elders with dementia		
divalproic acid (Depakote)	125-500 mg once or twice a day	Somnolence, dizziness,falls, orthostatic hypotension, increased confusion, & liver toxicity *all patients receiving this medication must have routine monitoring of Liver functioning and Depakote levels

Chapter 8 References

AARP. (2006). The pocket guide to staying healthy at 50+. Publication No. 04-1P001-A. Retrieved September 10, 2006, from www.ahrq.gov

About.com. (2010). MRI and Alzheimer's disease. Retrieved February 28, 2010, from http://alzheimers.about.com/lw/Health-Medicine/Conditions-and-diseases/MRIs-and-Alzheimers-Disease.htm

Alzheimer's Association. (2010). About Alzheimer's disease. Retrieved February 10, 2010, from www.alz.org

Alzheimer's disease facts and figures. (2009). Retrieved February 28, 2010, from http://www.alz.org/national/documents/summary_alzfactsfigures2009.pdf

Alzheimer's disease Research (2010). Retrieved February 21, 2010, from http://www.ahaf.org/alzhesimers/about/understanding/brain-nerve-cells.html

Alzheimer's Society. (2010). Alzheimer's disease: Risk factors. Retrieved February 28, 2010, from http://www.alzheimer.ca/english/disease/causes-riskfac.htm

AMHC (2007). Anxiety disorders in the elderly. Retrieved December 28, 2010, from http://www.healthyplace.com/anxiety-panic/main/anxiety-in-the-elderly/menu-id-69

Byrd, L. (2003). Terminal dementia in the elderly: awareness leads to more appropriate care. *Advance for Nurse Practitioners*. 11(9):65-72.

Cora, V. (2001) Elder Health. Community Health Nursing: Caring for the Public's Health. New York: Jones & Bartlett. p. 792-825.

Crystal, H. (2009). Dementia with Lewy Bodies. eMedicine Retrieved May 21, 2010, from http://emedicine.medscape.com/article/1135041-overview

Drugs.com (2010). FDA Approves the First Treatment for Dementia of Parkinson's Disease. Retrieved April 2, 2010, from http://www.drugs.com/news/fda-approves-first-dementia-parkinson-s-1842.html

eHow. (2010). Anxiety Medications Used in the Elderly with Dementia. Retrieved March 26, 2010, from http://www.ehow.com/facts_5761746_anxiety-medications-used-elderly-dementia.html

eMedicine. (2010). Parkinson's disease dementia. Retrieved April 2, 2010, from http://www.emedicinehealth.com/parkinson_disease_dementia/page3_em.htm

FamilyDoctor.org (2010). Memory Loss With Aging: What's Normal, What's Not. Retrieved May 21, 2010, from http://familydoctor.org/online/famdocen/home/seniors/common-older/124.html

HelpGuide. (2010). Lewy Body dementia. Retrieved March 31, 2010, from http://www.helpguide.org/elder/lewy_body_disease.htm

HelpGuide. (2010). Parkinson's disease dementia. Retrieved April 2, 2010, from http://www.helpguide.org/elder/parkinsons_disease.htm

HelpGuide. (2010). Pick's disease. Retrieved April 3, 2010, from http://www. helpguide.org/elder/picks_disease.htm

Hitti, M. (2006). FDA approves drug to treat Parkinson's dementia. Retrieved March 31, 2010, from http://www.webmd.com/parkinsons-disease/ news/20060628/fda-oks-drug-parkinsons-dementia

Keefer, A. (2010). How to Recognize the Symptoms of Anxiety in the Elderly | eHow.com Retrieved December 28, 2010, from http://www.ehow.com/ how_2202544_recognize-symptoms-anxiety-elderly.html#ixzz19T21OZy0

Kennard, C. (2006). Clock Drawing Test. Retrieved February 28, 2010, from http://alzheimers.about.com/od/diagnosisissues/a/clock_test.htm

Lindsay, J., Laurin, D., Verreault, R., Hébert, R., Helliwell, B., Hill G., & McDowell, I. (2002). Risk factors for Alzheimer's disease: a prospective analysis from the Canadian Study of Health and Aging. *American Journal of Epidemiology.* 156(5):445-53.

MayoClinic. (2006) Aging: What to expect as you get older. Retrieved October 14, 2006, from http://www.mayoclinic.com/health/aging/HA00040

Mayo Clinic. (2010) Alzheimer's stages: How the disease progresses. Retrieved February 27, 2010, from http://www.mayoclinic.com/health/ alzheimers-stages/AZ00041

Mayo Clinic. (2010). Alzheimer's disease: Diagnosing. Retrieved February 28, 2010, from http://www.mayoclinic.org/alzheimers-disease/diagnosis.html

Mayo Clinic. (2010). Alzheimer's disease: Risk factors. Retrieved February 28, 2010, from http://www.mayoclinic.com/health/alzheimers-disease/ DS00161/DSECTION=risk-factors

Mayo Clinic. (2010). Parkinson's disease. Retrieved March 31, 2010, from http://www.mayoclinic.com/health/parkinsons-disease/DS00295

Mayo Clinic. (2010). Vascular Dementia. Retrieved March 31, 2010, from http://www.mayoclinic.com/health/vascular-dementia/DS00934

MedicineNet. (2010). Dementia. Retrieved February 28, 2010, from http://www.medicinenet.com/dementia/article.htm

MedicineNet. (2010). What is Dementia? Retrieved March 29, 2010, from http://www.medicinenet.com/dementia/page2.htm

Medline Plus. (2010). Aging changes in the nervous system. Retrieved February 21, 2010, from http://www.nlm.nih.gov/medlineplus/ency/ article/004023.htm

Medscape. (2010). Alzheimer's disease: Pathology and Pathophysiology. Retrieved February 27, 2010, from http://www.medscape.com/ viewarticle/553256_2

Medscape. (2001). Quetiapine Improves Symptoms of Parkinson's Disease. Retrieved April 2, 2010, from http://www.medscape.com/ viewarticle/411260

Merck Manual. (2010). Dementia. Retrieved April 2, 2010, from http://www. merck.com/mmhe/sec06/ch083/ch083c.html#sec06-ch083-ch083c-541n

Miller, K., Zylstra, R., & Standridge, J. (2000). The geriatric patient: A systemic approach to maintaining health. *American Family Physician*. 61(4):1089-1106.

National Institute on Aging. (2010). Alzheimer's disease Fact Sheet. Retrieved May 21, 2010, from http://www.nia.nih.gov/Alzheimers/Publications/adfact.htm

Peterson, A. (2004). New Treatments For Alzheimer's Symptoms: To Curb Aggression, Paranoia In Dementia Patients, Doctors Turn to Schizophrenia Drugs. *The Wall Street Journal*. Retrieved March 26, 2010, from http://www.globalaging.org/health/us/2004/alz.htm

Pollock, B. (2007). SSRI Comparable to Antipsychotic for Psychosis in Dementia. *American Journal of Geriatric Psychiatry*. Retrieved April 2, 2010, from http://www.medpagetoday.com/Geriatrics/Dementia/6632

Reuben, D., Yoshikawa, T. & Besdine, R. (2003). What Is A Geriatric Syndrome Anyway? *Journal of the American Geriatrics Society.* 51(4):574-576.

Rosack, J. (2002). SSRI Improves Behavior Symptoms In Demented Elderly Patients. *Psychiatric News*. 37(7). p 28.

Salzman, C., Schneider, L., & Alexopoulos, G. (2010). Pharmacological Treatment of Depression in Late Life. Retrieved March 28, 2010, from http://www.acnp.org/g4/GN401000141/CH.html

Swanberg, M. & Kalapatapu, R. (2010). Parkinson Disease Dementia: Treatment & Medication. Medscape. Retrieved April 2, 2010, from http://emedicine.medscape.com/article/289595-treatment

Senior Journal. (2006). Beers Criteria for mediations to avoid in the elderly. Retrieved October 14, 2006, from http://seniorjournal.com/NEWS/Eldercare/3-12-08Beers.htm

Tangalos, E. (2010). Diagnosing Alzheimer's disease: From a Mayo Clinic Expert. Retrieved February 19, 2010, from http://www.mayoclinic.com/health/alzheimers/AZ00017

WebMD. (2010). Alzheimer's disease and other forms of Dementia. Retrieved February 27, 2010, from http://www.webmd.com/alzheimers/guide/alzheimers-dementia

WebMD. (2010). Down's syndrome and Alzheimer's disease. Retrieved February 28, 2010, from http://www.webmd.com/alzheimers/guide/alzheimers-down-syndrome

WebMD. (2010). Making the Diagnosis of Alzheimer's disease. Retrieved February 28, 2010, from http://www.webmd.com/alzheimers/guide/making-diagnosis?page=3

Wikipedia. (2010). MMSE. Retrieved February 28, 2010, from http://en.wikipedia.org/wiki/Mini-mental_state_examination#Interpretation

Chapter 9

Living Abilities

Self-sufficiency and the ability to take care of oneself greatly impacts the ability to be (or stay) independent. Physical as well as psychiatric problems can lead to an inability to perform the basic activities of daily living (ADLs) such as personal hygiene, dressing, eating, transferring from bed to chair, voluntary control of urine and fecal discharge, elimination, and moving around. Instrumental ADLs also affect the degree of independence a person is capable of managing, which includes doing light housework, preparing meals, taking medications, shopping for groceries or clothes, managing money, and using technology. This chapter will discuss factors affecting an elder's ability to maintain independence.

~

Aging takes a toll on many individuals and many elders have medical conditions which can impair a person's ability to care themselves and live independently. There is variability on the effects of aging among older individuals and there will be many factors which affect how well one ages. Each individual will experience some degree of anticipated declines in certain areas, such as cardiovascular function, muscle mass and bone strength, cognition and brain functioning. Other factors which affect how an individual ages that must be considered include environment, heredity factors, dietary intake, and the number and availability of social support systems.

Although changes occur with aging, individuals can do certain things to improve functioning and increase their chances of remaining independent. There is a great deal of evidence supporting the benefits of lifestyle interventions, specifically diet and physical activity, to assist many older individuals in overcoming the physical changes that occur with age and improve overall health, as well as quality of life (Kane et al, 2009). With regards to diet, eating foods low in saturated fats and a diet high in fresh fruits and vegetables offers some protective effects. Diet combined with regular physical exercise of 30 minutes daily has been shown to improve physical as well as mental health. And learning new knowledge and learning different skills will exercise the mind and preserve cognition.

SELF-RELIANCE

There are many issues to consider in order for elders to maintain independence and self-reliance, as well as be able to care for themselves. There are two domains to consider: physical limitations and cognitive limitations. Often, the ability to physically manage and care for oneself will be related to how rapidly fatigue occurs with physical exertion (heart and lung disease), ability to manipulate things and ambulate (arthritis and/or strokes), and ability to move around, both within one's environment (arthritis, as well as sensory deficits – vision, hearing, & balance) as well as getting to places beyond walking distance (driving ability, as well as cognitive problems). Health promotion and managing chronic diseases will assist in decreasing fatigue and increasing physical independence. Ambulation is discussed in-depth in chapter 2 on 'Falls' which takes into account vision, hearing, balance, arthritis, medications, and other issues affecting a person's ability to maneuver by themselves. The ability to feed oneself and issues surrounding eating are discussed in-depth in chapter 5 – Eating & Nutrition. Later in this chapter, some of the other issues will be discussed, including mobility outside the home (including driving and factors affecting self-care, such as bathing and grooming).

The ability to manage ADLs and IADLs are basic to caring for oneself and maintaining independence. The following are a list of these activities.

Basic Activities of Daily Living (ADLs)
- Eating (Feeding)
- Dressing
- Walking (Ambulation) as well as transferring from bed to chair or toilet
- Toileting and Continence
- Bathing & Grooming
- Communication

Instrumental Activities of Daily Living (IADLs)
- Writing
- Reading
- Cooking
- Cleaning
- Shopping
- Doing laundry
- Climbing stairs
- Using the telephone
- Managing medication
- Managing money
- Ability to work
- Ability to travel

Promoting Healthy Behaviors
Healthy Older Adults are encouraged to follow a few guidelines to maintain and enhance health:

Overall
- Stay physically active
- Avoid mental distress
- Perform good oral hygiene (brush & floss teeth)
- Minimize the complications of physical disabilities

Diet & Exercise
- Include leisure time physical activity
- Eat 5+ fruits & vegetables daily
- If overweight – lose weight
- If smoking – STOP

Preventive health measures
- Annual Flu shot
- Pneumonia Vaccine – at least once (or every 10 years)
- Mammogram every 2 years
- Have a screening colonoscopy

- Have cholesterol checked at least every 5 years (preferably annually)
- Annual vision assessment
- Annual dental check-up

Other screening tests

- Women: Pap smear every 3 years up to the age of 65
    o more often if there is a history of pelvic/uterine cancer
- Men: PSA blood work annually up to the age of 70
    o more often if there is a history of prostate cancer
- Consider screening for Osteoporosis if one is at risk, there is a history of fractures, or one is on certain medications

Maintaining Health

- Know what conditions all medications are being taken to treat
- Bring ALL MEDICATIONS to the office/clinic visits EVERY TIME
- Remember to take medications as prescribed and tell someone if there are problems caused by a medication
- Annual check-ups and as dictated depending upon health status and conditions

Factors Affecting Ability to Live Independently

An older person's ability to live independently depends on their ability to care for self and maneuver within their environment. It is also dependent on a person's ability to obtain the necessary living items, such as food and medications. Factors which affect an individual's ability to do these things can be related to physical and/or mental capacities, including the following systems/problems:

Table 9-1. *Sensory Changes with Aging*	
NORMAL AGING CHANGES AFFECTING AN OLDER PERSON'S ABILITY TO BE INDEPENDENT *Not all elders will experience all of these changes, but many will be affected by these common changes due to normal aging processes.*	
Vision: All elders experience some degree of decline in vision	• <u>Depth perception</u>: The cornea, the part of the eye which refracts light, becomes flatter, less smooth, and thicker making older eyes more susceptible to astigmatism. These changes can affect the ability to judge distance, including judging the speed of oncoming traffic. • <u>Decreased ability to differentiate colors</u>: There is a yellowing of the lens which causes some reduction of the eye's ability to discriminate blues, greens, and violets; colors seen more clearly are yellows, oranges, reds, and black. • <u>Ptosis</u>: An older person can have loose skin on the lids of the eye. Eyelids may droop as elasticity is lost, causing the person's visual field to be diminished. • <u>Dry Eyes</u>: There can be a decrease in orbicular muscle strength causing the eyelid to stay open slightly, which can lead to corneal dryness. • <u>Presbyopia</u>: After 40 years of age, a person's eye looses the ability to adjust to close objects and this problem continues to progress throughout life, leading to a progressive farsightedness. • <u>Decreased Peripheral Vision</u>: Peripheral vision decreases, making the visual field smaller (a person can no longer see things approaching from the side as readily).

(CONTINUED)

Vision: *(CONTINUED)*	• <u>Slower Pupil Accommodation</u>: Pupil size is smaller, creating a slower constriction in the presence of bright light. There is a slowing of the pupil's dilation in dark settings and a slowing in the ability to accommodate to changes in light. Older eyes need three times more light, making night vision somewhat impaired in older adults. Glare occurs more often for elders. For example, sunlight may be reflected off shiny objects or there may be a glare around headlights of cars. • <u>Glaucoma</u>: The anterior chamber of the eye decreases as the thickness of the lens increases. In some elders, there is an increase in the density of collagen fibers, leading to inefficient resorption of intraocular fluids and increased pressure in the eye – glaucoma. • <u>Cataracts</u>: Lens opacities can develop after the age of 50, causing cloudiness in vision; this can progress to obscure vision completely. • <u>Opacities</u>: can develop and can be seen as spots or clusters of dots in the visual field (which are coalesced vitreous that have broken off the periphery or central part of the retina). These are largely harmless, although they can be annoying. Drusen (yellow-white) spots can develop in an area of the macula and, as long as not accompanied with distortion of objects or a decrease in vision, this pigmentation is not clinically significant.

(CONTINUED)

Table 9-1. *Sensory Changes with Aging (CONTINUED)*

Hearing loss: Approximately 1/3 of elders have some degree of hearing impairment. It can occur gradually. Cues to a hearing problem when driving is inattention to sounds, such as honking, emergency sirens, or a child's bicycle bell.	• <u>Cerumen</u>: (Ear Wax): The Auditory canal narrows and the cerumen glands atrophy in older adults, causing thicker and dryer cerumen (ear wax) which makes its removal more difficult and can lead to blockage of the canal. • <u>Presbycusis</u>: (Hearing Loss): The tympanic membrane becomes dull, less flexible, retracted, and slightly gray in appearance. The ossicle joints between the malleus and stapes can become calcified and lead to a reduction in vibration of these bones and thus reduced sound transmission. There is a slight degeneration of the internal parts of the ear, which leads to impaired transmission of sound waves along the nerve pathways. These changes are considered the most common reason for hearing loss in elders. Another type of hearing loss is caused by atrophy of the organ of Corti which is sensory hearing loss. Loss of cochlear neurons can cause neural hearing loss. • <u>Tinnitis</u>: Sometimes there is an impairment of the otic nerve, which can lead to a constant or recurring high-pitched tinnitus, such as clicking, buzzing, roaring, or ringing sound, in one or both ears. Causes of this problem include medications, infections, or cerumen accumulation; a blow to the head can also cause this problem. Tinnitus can be more pronounced in quiet settings.

(CONTINUED)

Motor skills: Full range of motion and good muscle strength are crucial for safety in mobility and when an elder is on the road driving. Certain chronic conditions in elders can limit mobility. Illnesses such as rheumatoid arthritis, Parkinson's disease, sleep apnea, heart disease and diabetes can decrease flexibility and reaction time, raising the risks for accidents.	• <u>Loss of Strength</u>: Muscles, tendons, and joints can lose some strength and flexibility with aging, unless the person is physically active. These changes can lead to a slower reaction time in response to stimuli. For example, an elder may be at risk when driving if there is a need to stop quickly to avoid oncoming traffic but the individual is unable to react rapidly enough to avoid an accident. • <u>Decreased Range of Motion of the Neck</u>: Bone mass or density can diminish as bones lose calcium and other minerals, especially in women after menopause. The spine is made up of several bones which have a gel-like cushion between them. In aging, the disks gradually lose fluid and become thinner causing the spinal column to become curved and compressed, leading to kyphosis. Bone spurs can occur due to aging and overall use of the spine. The cumulative effect is decreased ability to turn one's head adequately.

Drowsiness or sleepiness: Certain medications can cause drowsiness. Additionally, some elders become tired during the day or have an increased tendency to doze off during the day.	• Certain medical conditions make an elder fatigue easily.
	• Medications that can cause drowsiness include:
	    o benzodiazapines
	    o some antihistamines
	    o certain glaucoma medications
	    o non-steroidal anti-inflammatory drugs
	    o muscle relaxants

(Aging Eyes 2006; Ebersole et al, 2004; Eye Digest, 2010; MedicineNet, 2006; Helpguide's Senior Driving: Risk Factors, Safety Tips and Transportation Options; Tumosa, 2000)

Sense	What to Assess	Potential Problems
Table 9-2. *Assessing for Potential Problems Due to Sensory Changes with Aging*		
Vision	Assess ability to watch television, read, drive, or perform any activity requiring eyesight	Inability to read or fails a vision test; i.e., Snellen chart assessment (Minimum to pass: 20/40)
Hearing	Assess ability to hear noises and/or speech (both high and low tones), as well as ability to comprehend what is being said (comprehension); i.e., the ability to appropriately answer questions and follow simple requests	Inability to hear and understand speech or fails hearing test in one or both ears (Minimum to pass: 1000Hz in one ear & 2000Hz in both ears)
Mobility	Assess the ability to get up from a seated position, walk 20 feet briskly, turn around and walk back, and then sit down again	Unable to complete this task in less than 15 seconds
Urinary Incontinence	Assess if there are any incontinence episodes in the past year; if so, how many episodes each week	Yes, to any episodes of incontinence

Sense	What to Assess	Potential Problems
Weight stability	Assess if there has been any unintentional weight loss over the past 6 months	Weight loss of 10 lbs in 6 months; or if person weighs less than 100 lbs, loss of 5 lbs in 6 months
Recent recall *i.e., short term memory*	Assess a person's ability to remember 3 items after 15 minutes (3-item recall)	Unable to recall all 3 items after 15 minutes
Depression	Assess for sadness, depression, or anxious symptoms	Yes to any of these items
Endurance	Assess for any of the following: 1. Unable to perform strenuous activity, such as fast walking or bicycling 2. Unable to perform heavy work such as housecleaning – washing windows, walls, or floors 3. Unable to shop for groceries or clothes due to physical or mental restrictions 4. Unable to get to places that are beyond walking distance 5. Unable to bath self – either sponge bath or shower 6. Unable to dress self by putting on a shirt, pants – buttoning and zipping, as well as putting on shoes	The individual is disabled if unable to do any of the listed items

(Moore & Sui, 1996)

Functional Status

The functional status of an older individual is defined as the capacity to safely perform ADLs and IADLs and is a good indicator of health as well as illness. Some functional decline may be prevented or diminished with prompt and aggressive intervention, such as walking ability, toileting schedules, enhanced communication, adaptive equipment, and attention to health (which includes diet, activity, and use of medications to optimize health). Some functional decline may occur progressively and is not reversible. This decline often accompanies chronic disease states such as degenerative joint disease, Parkinson's disease, dementia, heart failure, and cancer (Hartford, 2011).

Functional status is influenced by changes due to normal aging as well as acute or chronic illness and the person's ability to adapt to their physical environment. A decline in an older person's functional abilities is often the initial symptom of acute illness like infections such as pneumonia and urinary tract infection. These declines are usually reversible but require medical evaluation (Hartford, 2011).

Factors which can affect an individual's functional status and place a person at risk for decline include injuries, acute illness, medication side effects, pain, depression, malnutrition, decreased mobility, prolonged bedrest (including the use of physical restraints), prolonged use of indwelling urinary catheters, and changes in a person's environment or routine. Complications of functional decline include loss of independence, falls, urinary and/or bowel incontinence, malnutrition, decreased socialization, depression, and increased risk for long-term institutionalization such as a nursing home (Hartford, 2011).

Restoration in function can also be a measure of return to health, such as for those individuals recovering from exacerbations of illnesses like cardiovascular or respiratory diseases and acute infections, recovering from joint replacement surgery, or new strokes. Functional status evaluation assists in planning future care needs of an older person after a hospitalization, including short-term skilled care in a nursing home and/or home care. A person's physical environment should be given attention to address any special needs to maintain and enhance function; i.e., chairs with arms, elevated toilet seat, levers versus door knobs, enhanced lighting (Hartford, 2011).

Improving Strength & Balance – *See chapter 2 on falls for Strength and Balance Improvement*
Ways to increase independence through altering how things are done or use of assistive devices:

Walking outdoors
- Use a walking stick, cane, or walker
- If the person has decreased ability to walk, Increase outgoing activities by encouraging the person to use a car or obtain a ride
- Walk with someone whose arm can be can used to steady oneself
- Get an electric scooter

Standing for a period
- Take frequent breaks to sit down and rest
- Get higher stool to perch
- Alter worktops to be the right height when sitting
- Delegate the task to someone else

Strength in hands
- To strengthen grip – look for gadgets in shops, such as squeeze balls, vices, etc
- Have things or gadgets delivered by mail order
- Only buy items that can be opened easily
- Ask someone to do these things

Stairs
- Only go up/down once a day
- Move to a one story house/apartment
- Get handrail(s) fitted
- Get a stair-lift
- Live downstairs
- Getting in/out of the bath
- Fit grab rails by bath
- Get a seat to go in the bathtub – make sure the seat has suction cups to prevent it from moving and causing a fall

- Consider installing a special bath
- Replace bathtub with walk-in shower
- Getting up/sitting down
- Put extra cushion on seat or chair
- Get new, higher chair
- Get electrically operated riser/recliner
- Ask medical provider or social services for advice

(Sayer, 2007)

MANEUVERING OUTSIDE ONE'S OWN HOME - DRIVING
Weighing the Risks (Safety) against the Benefits (an Individual's Independence & Autonomy) of Driving

Safety trumps autonomy when circumstances are evident that an older person and others are at risk (or in danger) due to compromised driving abilities. But when the threat is not absolutely clear that there is a significant problem for an individual and the family's wishes (that the person not drive due to safety concerns) differ from the individual's wishes (to continue to drive based on a desire for autonomy, independence, and control), conflict is inevitable. Moreover, the consequences to the older person of giving up driving are not trivial and the burdens imposed by loss of the driving privileges, as well as loss of independence, are both practical and psychological. For individuals who may be isolated from others, whether living in rural or suburban environments, a personal automobile may be the only readily available means of transportation. In urban areas, there may be public transportation, taxi or car services available, but many elders are not familiar (or comfortable) with using this type of transportation and may find it confusing. Relying on others for transportation is not always a welcome solution for many elders, even if it is provided by family or friends. Convincing an older individual to retire from driving for 'safety's sake' will sometimes have undesirable consequences, including rebellion by an elder or an argument (Kennedy, 2009).

Warning Signs for Older Drivers

Use the Warning Signs for Older Drivers to help families and caregivers better understand when an individual's ability to drive is becoming unsafe and there is decline in an individual's abilities as the disease progresses.

- Consider the frequency and severity of incidents
  - o Several minor incidents or an unusual, major incident may require immediate action
- Look for patterns of change over time
  - o Isolated or minor incidents may not require immediate or drastic action
- Avoid an alarming reaction
  - o Take notes and have conversations at a later, convenient time

Share observations with the individual, family members, and caregivers. Families need to consider the circumstances and seriousness of unsafe driving practices before deciding the next steps which should be taken – choices include:

1. continue monitoring the elder's driving
2. modify the elder's driving
3. have the elder stop driving immediately

How can an Elder Driver be evaluated when safety is a concern?

When there is suspicion that an individual might be an unsafe driver, close monitoring is essential before a definitive decision should be made, whether it is time to limit driving or give up the driver's license altogether. Some steps include:

- Watch for changes in driving habits, general behavior, and health issues which could affect driving
- Encourage a driving evaluation through the local Department of Motor Vehicles, along with refresher driving lessons; AARP encourages a "Driver Safety Course" for elders who are having problems with driving

Steps to Stopping Driving or 'Taking the Keys'

Identify the Problem: It begins with admitting an individual's driving is an issue:

1. Assess an Individual's driving abilities
2. Ride along and observe
3. Have a friend or another relative ride along and observe
4. Have the Person meet someone who can observe the person's driving abilities:
   - Make sure the observer arrives prior to the person who is being evaluated

- The observer should be positioned to watch the driver's arrival
- The observer should be sure to have the person navigate an intersection – preferably have the person cross/turn at a stop sign
- Watch for use of blinkers

5. Watch for appropriateness of stopping
   <u>Problems</u>: *Stopping too far back from the line or in the middle of the intersection*

6. Watch ability in crossing intersection with other traffic
   <u>Problems</u>: *hesitation to enter intersection or entering the intersection out of turn*

7. Watch the person park
   <u>Problems</u>: *parking too close to other vehicles, parking too far into space or too far back*

REMEMBER SAFETY: *Time of day is important – do not perform the evaluation at evening or night-time; aim for light traffic times, and good weather*

1. Identify State laws and restrictions on Individual Drivers with Physical Handicaps, as well as Drivers with a diagnosis of dementia

2. Enlist the Individual Driver in discussions about stopping driving

3. Keep a driving log to document problems
   - Drives too slowly
   - Stops in traffic for no reason or ignores traffic signs
   - Becomes lost on a familiar route
   - Lacks good judgment
   - Has difficulty with turns, lane changes, or highway exits
   - Drifts into other lanes of traffic or drives on the wrong side of the street
   - Signals incorrectly or does not signal
   - Has difficult seeing pedestrians, objects, or other vehicles
   - Falls asleep while driving or gets drowsy
   - Parks inappropriately
   - Gets ticketed for traffic violations
   - Is increasingly nervous or irritated when driving
   - Has accidents, near misses, or "fender benders"

4. Decrease the person's need to drive and/or limit driving
   - Have groceries, meals, and prescriptions delivered to the home
   - Arrange for a barber or hairdresser to make home visits – or – go to the hairdresser together
   - Invite friends and family over for regular visits
   - Arrange for family and friends to take the individual on social outings

5. When the time comes for the person to stop driving: Discuss your observations with the person – use the driving log (the list of reasons why the person is not safe to continue driving); if the discussion becomes heated, this will assist in your ability to make your points
6. Suggest alternatives to driving

Easing the Transition from Driving

One of the most difficult tasks for families to accomplish is transitioning an individual from driving. But family members must balance the needs and safety of their loved ones against the safety of the community in which they live. The most effective approach to limit or stop a person from driving involves developing a plan and will probably include a combination of strategies that fit the person's circumstances, resources, and relationships. For many older individuals, it may be a better approach to reduce the person's frequency of driving over time rather than stopping it abruptly. Attention should be given to meeting a person's day-to-day needs, including obtaining food, medications, and medical needs. It is also important to address a person's social needs. Whenever possible, include the elder in planning ahead to limit and eventually stop driving.

In some cases of severe physical impairment or cognitive impairment, individuals with dementia may realize there is a problem and begin limiting where and when they drive. The following signs indicate that a person with dementia is modifying their driving behaviors:

- Drives only short distances
- Drives only to familiar places
- Avoids difficult situations
- Avoids driving at night, in heavy traffic, on heavily traveled roads and/or during bad weather

Keep in mind that driving even short distances during daylight hours and in good weather can pose a risk if the person's driving skills are impaired. Most accidents have been reported to occur close to home (Hartford, 2010).

Enough is Enough, Driving MUST be Stopped

Sometimes an individual with physical impairments that present a safety hazard, or those with a diagnosis of dementia, should be 'stopped' from driving over his/her objections. It might be very difficult for families to come to this decision, especially if the individual is very independent. However, the safety of the person and the safety of others must come first. An unsafe driver can seriously injure or kill themselves or others. If appropriate evaluations and recommendations have been made, it has been determined that driving is no longer safe, and rational discussions with the person have not been successful in persuading a person to stop driving, then creativity in finding a solution is necessary. This can be a difficult task and each situation requires an individualized plan. In some cases, there is a need to take further actions, such as taking away the car keys, selling or disabling the vehicle, and/or enlisting authority figures (including healthcare providers or the local police) to assist in explaining the importance of safe driving and the legal implications of unsafe driving (HelpGuide, 2010).

Legal Restrictions for Elder Drivers

A person's age is not a sufficient basis for losing a driver's license or even for a person to be mandated to undergo re-examination for a driver's license. Older individuals do not automatically lose their driving privileges and/or drivers license with physical impairments or a diagnosis of dementia, because they have certain legal rights. State Departments of Motor Vehicles (DMV) do have the authority to investigate and re-examine any individual who demonstrates a potential risk of driving dangerously due to physical, psychiatric, or behavioral problems, or there is evidence of poor driving record.

State-by-state Regulations on Elderly Drivers License Renewal

- Six states (Florida, Maine, Oregon, South Carolina, Utah, and Virginia) and the District of Columbia require elderly drivers (age varies from state to state-from 55 to 70) to take a vision test. drivers to take a vision test when renewing a license

- Another way states monitor older drivers is by no longer permitting drivers over a certain age to renew their licenses by mail
  - Five states (Alaska, California, Colorado, Louisiana, and Montana) restrict mail renewals and online renewal. Age varies from state to state– from 61 to 70
  - Two states (Illinois and New Hampshire) require a road test if the driver is 75 years old or older

State legal requirements to report an unsafe driver

- All state Departments of Motor Vehicles, Highway Safety, or Transportation have an office where a family member or healthcare provider can make a referral about an unsafe driver
  - The state DMV office will investigate the claim to determine if the driver should be mandated to take a road test in order to maintain his/her license
- In California, however, healthcare providers are required to submit a confidential report of individuals who have a diagnosis of dementia

  'This information is forwarded to the Department of Motor Vehicles (DMV), which is authorized to take action against the driving privileges of any individual who is unable to safely operate a motor vehicle. If the physician's report indicates that an individual has moderate or severe dementia, that individual will no longer be permitted to operate a motor vehicle. DMV has determined that only drivers with dementia in the mild stages may still have the cognitive functions necessary to continue driving safely. DMV requires re-examination for all individuals reported to have mild dementia.'   Family Caregiver Alliance, (2010)

- Compared to other medical issues which affect driving abilities: In California, Delaware, Nevada, New Jersey, Oregon, and Pennsylvania, healthcare providers are required to report individuals with a diagnosis of epilepsy

California DMV Procedure in Management of Individuals with Dementia
The California DMV follows specific procedures when a medical report regarding an individual with dementia is received:

1. A computer search is conducted to locate the individual's name, verify that he/she has a license, and examine the person's driving history
2. The individual is contacted by letter and sent a "Driver Medical Evaluation" form to authorize the primary healthcare provider to submit medical information about the status of the dementia, including the person's cognitive functioning
3. A Driver Safety hearing officer reviews the medical form: If the person

is in the mild stage of dementia, the individual is scheduled for a re-examination with DMV; if the individual is in the later stages of dementia, their driving privileges will be revoked; and if the individual fails to submit medical documentation within the requested time frame, all driving privileges will be suspended.

4. A re-examination is completed, involving three phases: a visual test, a written test, and an interview.

   - Visual Test: Effective January 1, 2001, all drivers must have corrected visual acuity of better than 20/200 in the better eye without the use of a bioptic telescope
   - Written Test: The individual is given the standard DMV written examination designed to test an individual's knowledge of the road. The written test allows the DMV office to determine not only the person's knowledge of driving laws, but also mental competency and cognitive skills
   - Interview: An in-person interview focuses on the medical documentation as well as the driver's ability to coherently answer questions about his/her health, medical treatment, driving record, need to drive, daily routine, need for assistance with daily activities, etc. Persons who do well up to this point are then given a driving test. Those who do poorly on the visual, written, or verbal tests may have their driving privilege suspended or revoked.

5. The driving test is designed to test driving skills that might be affected by dementia. Initially, the person is observed to identify if the individual can find his/her car. Then, the examiner gives a series of commands, rather than one direction at a time (for example, "Please drive to the corner, turn left and turn right at the first street"). The test generally lasts longer than the ordinary driver's test in order to gauge whether or not fatigue is a problem.

6. If the individual passes the driving test, the license is generally not suspended or revoked, although restrictions may be imposed on the license, such as no freeway driving, no night driving, or driving allowed only within a certain radius. DMV may want to review the individual's driving skills again in six to twelve months. At that time, the entire process is repeated.

7. An appeals process is available if the individual or family wishes to contest the suspension or revocation of the driver's license. At the hearing, the individual may present evidence, such as new medical information, to prove that the dementia does not impair his or her ability to safely operate a motor vehicle.

8. DMV can provide a California identification card to those persons who will no longer have a driver's license.

(Family Caregiver Alliance, 2010)

Alternatives to Driving

Asking an individual to stop driving can be a delicate issue. Be prepared when the person asks how they will get around or get the things they need. Have a plan and the appropriate answers prepared.

Let Others Do the Driving – explore all transportation options – from public transportation to informal arrangements with families, friends, and support groups.

Public Transportation – this is an option if the individual can maneuver this type of transportation and it is accessible for the person.

Pay-for-service Transportation – Taxis can be a cost-effective alternative, especially when fares are compared to the expense of gas, insurance, taxes, repairs and car payments. Taxis could also be used for people in middle to later stages of dementia if:

- There are no behavioral problems and the driver can be given explicit directions
- In the moderate to advanced stages of dementia, someone may need to be available to meet the person at the beginning and end of the trip

Some taxi companies will set up accounts for family caregivers so a person with dementia has easy access to transportation without worrying about payment.

Friends and Relatives – or caregivers can offer to drive the individual with dementia to appointments or social events. Families will be more likely to assist with driving if the primary caregiver makes specific requests and schedules appointments at times that work for those requested to help.

Co-Piloting Is <u>Not</u> a Good Solution – Some families or caregivers act as co-pilots to keep an individual driving longer, giving directions and instructions on how to drive. Although this strategy may work for a limited time, it can be hazardous and there is rarely enough time for some elderly drivers to foresee the danger and respond quickly enough to avoid an accident.

Early Planning to Limit Driving

When possible, include the individual with dementia in discussions surrounding driving safety and future plans to cease driving. It is better to obtain the person's input and understand their point of view while conveying how the person's health issues may eventually affect the person's ability to drive. It is better to this discussion with someone while the person can still understand these reasons and why this decision will be necessary; this allows the person to understand the rational arguments for safety. This method respects the individual's dignity by focusing on how the medical issues affect the person and their abilities to drive safely as the reason for driving restrictions and cessation, instead of implying that the individual is any lesser a person.

Build Social Support to reduce stress and increase chances for success. Encourage the person to increase the use of others to meet the needs the person would normally meet through driving. Relying on others for emotional support, transportation assistance, and financial help or to meet other needs are good alternatives. For example, a child or neighbor might be able to run an errand or pay a visit; a long-distance relative might be willing to pay for an occasional driver or taxi; or a friend might be able to observe driving ability and habits.

Other Opportunities to Limit Driving

With some foresight and planning, families may be able to create non-confrontational ways to make driving less appealing or less necessary. Some examples include:

- When an individual with a diagnosis of dementia is moving to an area that has more support services, discuss alternative transportation in the new location – particularly because these individuals may be more uncomfortable and at higher risk of accidents when driving in unfamiliar places (Relocation may help encourage the individual to limit or stop driving).
- Families may be able to use discussions surrounding financial issues to build a case for selling the car by itemizing the many costs of operating a vehicle including upkeep, taxes, tag, gasoline, and insurance costs.
- Physical changes which affect driving may be used as an excuse to limit or stop driving (see physical changes listed earlier in this chapter).

Chapter 9 References

Aging Eyes (2006). Retrieved April 4, 2010, from http://www.agingeye.net

Dobbs, A. R. (1997). "Evaluating the Driving Competence of Dementia Patients." *Alzheimer's Disease and Associated Dementia*. Vol. 11, Suppl: 8-12.

Ebersole, Hess, & Luggen (2004). Toward Healthy Aging. 6th ed. Mosby, Inc: Philadelphia.

ElderGym. (2011). Elder Strength Training. Retrieved April 1, 2011, from http://www.eldergym.com/elderly-strength.html; http://www.eldergym.com/elderly-balance.html

Family Caregiver Alliance. (2010). Dementia, Driving, and California State Law. Retrieved April 4, 2010, from http://www.caregiver.org/caregiver/jsp/content_node.jsp?nodeid=433

Hartford Foundation (2000). At the Crossroads: A Guide to Alzheimer's Disease, Dementia, and Driving. Retrieved April 4, 2010, from http://www.thehartford.com/alzheimers

Hartford Foundation. (2010). Family discussions about Alzheimer's disease, dementia, and driving. Retrieved April 2, 2010, from http://www.thehartford.com/alzheimers

HelpGuide. (2010). Helpguide's Senior Driving: Risk Factors, Safety Tips and Transportation Options. Retrieved April 4, 2010, from http://beta.helpguide.org/elder/senior_citizen_driving.htm

Kane, R., Ouslander, J., Abrass, I., & Resnick, B. (2009) Essentials of Clinical Geriatrics. 6th ed. McGraw Hill Medical: New York.

Kennedy, G. (2009). Psychogeriatrics: Advanced Age, Dementia, and Driving. *Psychiatric Weekly*. 4(18). Retrieved April 3, 2010, from http://www.psychiatryweekly.com/aspx/article/articledetail.aspx?articleid=984

Kresevic, D. (2011). FUNCTION: Nursing Standard of Practice Protocol: Assessment of Function in Acute Care. Hartford: ConsultGeriRN.org Retrieved April 1, 2011, from http://consultgerirn.org/topics/function/want_to_know_more

LA 4 Seniors.com (2001). Dangerous Driving and Seniors. Retrieved April 1, 2011, from http://www.la4seniors.com/driving.htm

Mayo Foundation for Medical Education and Research (2001). Dementia: Should Your Patient be Driving? Retrieved April 1, 2011, from http://www.mayo.edu/geriatrics-rst/driving.html

MedicineNet (2006). Hearing loss and aging. Retrieved October 14, 2006, from http://www.medicinenet.com/script/main/art.asp?articlekey=20432

Moore, A., & Sui, A. (1996). Screening for common problems in ambulatory elderly: clinical confirmation of a screening instrument. *American Journal of Medicine*. (100). 438-443.

Sayer, A. (2007). Readiness of elders to use assistive devices to maintain their independence in the home. *Age and Ageing*. 36(4); 465-467.

Tumosa, N. (2000). Aging and the eye. Merck manual of geriatrics. Whitehouse Station, NJ. Merck research Laboratories.

Chapter 10

Skin Integrity

There are many changes to the integumentary system (the skin) which can adversely affect older individuals. There are many factors that can cause the skin to be more fragile, tear easily, and heal more slowly. This chapter will review the changes which can lead to problems, including skin tears, shingles, fungal infections, cellulitis, and ulcerations. A management protocol will be presented to care for common skin problems in elders.

Skin is the body's first line of defense from bacteria. There are a number of changes in the skin of elders that occur due to the aging process. And there are a number of skin issues in older adults. Sunlight is a major cause of the skin changes that occur with normal aging – changes such as wrinkles, dryness, and age spots. For example, an older person usually sweats less, leading to difficulty regulating body temperature. There is oil production by the skin, leading to increased dryness. There is oil production by the skin, leading to increased dryness., leading to increased dryness. As the skin ages, it becomes thinner and loses fat, so it looks less plump and smooth. Underlying structures – veins and bones in particular – become more prominent. A break in the skin can take longer to heal. A person can delay these changes by staying out of the sun. Although nothing can completely undo sun damage, the skin does have the ability to repair itself. So, it's never too late to protect an individual's skin from the harmful effects of the sun.

AGING CHANGES TO SKIN

- Skin thins with time
  - o Dermis loses 20% thickness
  - o Becomes less elastic and more fragile, with an increase in bruising
  - o Slower wound healing by 33%
- Increased melatonin synthesis
  - o Increase skin pigmentation/aging spots

- Reduction in dermal blood vessels
- Deceased production of natural oils causing skin
  o Drier
  o Wrinkles
- Perspire less
- Nerve Density decreases/Sensory Activity decreases
- Hair may gray and thin
- Unwanted hair production
  o Women – Chin
  o Men – Ears
- Nail Changes
  o Grow at about half the pace as when younger
  o Nails may become thicker and more brittle
  o Skin tags are common

SKIN PROBLEMS COMMON IN OLDER ADULTS

- corns and calluses
- pruritis (itching)
- rosacea
- psoriasis
- onychomycosis
- dermatitis (rashes)
  o seborrheic
  o contact
  o fungal/candidiasis
- actinic keratoses
- neoplasms (skin cancers)
  o squamous
  o basal
  o melanoma
- cellulitis (infections)
- lower extremity ulcers
- senile purpura
- herpes zoster or shingles
- burns
- pressure ulcers
- skin tears
- bruising

(Mayo Clinic, 2010; eMedicineNet.com, 2010; GNRS, 2007; Touhy & Jett, 2010)

SKIN CANCER

Skin cancer is the most common type of cancer in the United States, with evidence that 40 to 50% of individuals over 65 will have some form of skin cancer in their lifetime. Annual assessment of skin should be done to assess for changes in skin, any new lesions, or changes in long standing lesions for all older individuals. Potential clues to a problem with a skin lesion include bleeding, darkening, increase in size, or change in appearance. Evaluation by a skin specialist, such as a dermatologist, may be necessary for any suspicious lesion that does not resolve with initial treatment (GNRS, 2007).

Ways to promote skin health and to prevent skin cancer include:
- Avoid sun exposure, especially between 10 a.m. and 3 p.m.
- Use sunscreen
- Wear protective clothing
- Avoid artificial tanning
- Check skin often for discolorations and any change in moles
- Use lotions to moisturize skin
- Avoid traumatizing skin
- If skin tears easily, keep it moisturized and cover open skin areas promptly, apply antibiotic ointment and band-aide or dressing until healed; consider wearing long-sleeved shirts and long pants to offer a barrier and prevent injury
- Take Vitamin E 400 IU daily
- If a sore or ulcer is present, consider Vitamin C 500 mg daily and a multivitamin with iron daily

SKIN PROBLEMS

Corns are the result of mechanical trauma to the skin due to a thickening of the outer layer of skin, also referred to as the epidermis. They are most commonly caused by friction and pressure between the bones of the foot and ill-fitting footwear and are a normal physiological response of the skin.

MANAGEMENT for a corn:
- Use over-the-counter pads to protect areas where corns and calluses develop.
- Be careful in the use of over-the-counter liquid corn removers or medicated corn pads; these contain salicylic acid, which may lead to an ulcer or infection of the area. This is especially problematic in elders with diabetes and poor circulation because it can irritate healthy skin and lead to infection.
- Soak the person's hands or feet in warm, soapy water to soften corns and calluses. This will make it easier to remove the thickened skin.

- Thin out thickened skin – during or after bathing, rub corns or calluses with a pumice stone or washcloth to help remove a layer of toughened skin. Don't use a pumice stone if an elderly person is diabetic because of the increased risk of infection. Whether or not an older individual has diabetes, don't cut or shave corns or calluses, because this could lead to an infection.
- Moisturize skin – apply moisturizer to the person's hands and feet to help keep skin soft. Elders should wear comfortable shoes, wear socks that are well-fitting, and wear cushioned shoes until a corn or callus disappears.
- Encourage the use of socks made of a polyester-cotton blend because they wick moisture away better than all-cotton socks do. Additionally, have the person wear socks that fit properly.

(Horne, 2007)

Pruritus is an itch (also referred to as urticaria) or a sensation that makes a person want to scratch. It can cause discomfort and be frustrating. If pruritus is severe, it can lead to sleeplessness, anxiety, agitation, and depression. The exact cause of the problem may be unknown. And it may be a complex process involving nerves that respond to certain chemicals like histamine that are released in the skin, or it can be related to the processing of nerve signals in the brain. Pruritus can be a part of skin diseases or internal disorders, or due to faulty processing of the itch sensation within the nervous system; any new onset of pruritus warrants investigation into the cause, so it can be properly treated. If there is no identifiable cause and it is diagnosed as IDIOPATHIC PRURITUS.

MANAGEMENT includes:

- When bathing or showering, use tepid or lukewarm water.
- Use mild cleansers with low pH. Rinse off soap film completely, pat the skin lightly, and immediately apply a moisturizing lotion or cream after bathing.
- Have the person wear light, loose clothing.
- A cool work or domestic environment can help reduce the severity of itching.
- And for itchy conditions where blistering or weeping of the skin is present, such as chicken pox or poison ivy, a cool oatmeal bath or topical drying agents (such as calamine lotion) can be helpful.

(Mayo Clinic, 2010; eMedicineNet.com, 2010; GNRS, 2007; Touhy & Jett, 2010)

Dermatitis is a general term that describes an inflammation of the skin. There are different types of dermatitis: seborrheic dermatitis, atopic dermatitis (eczema), and fungal dermatitis. Although dermatitis can have many causes and occur in many forms, it usually involves swollen, reddened and itchy skin. It is a common condition that usually isn't life-threatening or contagious. But, it can make an elderly person feel uncomfortable and self-conscious.

Seborrheic dermatitis is a common scalp and facial condition that often causes dandruff

TREATMENT:
- Shampoos that contain tar, pyrithione zinc, salicylic acid or ketoconazole as the active ingredient
  - Nizoral Shampoo
  - Selsun Blue shampoo
- Hydrocortisone creams and lotions for nonscalp seborrheic dermatitis
- 1% hydrocortisone cream twice a day
- Nonsteroidal medications, called immunomodulators (immunomodulators affect the immune system and have anti-inflammatory and mild antifungal properties)
  - tacrolimus (Protopic)
  - pimecrolimus (Elidel)

Contact dermatitis is a rash that results from either repeated contact with irritants or contact with allergy-producing substances, such as poison ivy
- Heat and scratching worsen the problem or increase the spread of the condition
  - Cool tepid water
  - Drying agents

MANAGEMENT:
- 1% hydrocortisone cream twice a day
- Avoid irritants
- Consider treatments for itch
- Presciption medications to consider include steroids

Fungal dermatitis - Skin fungus infections present with itching, flaking, redness, and thickened skin; this condition can look just like other types of dermatitis or skin allergy. The skin issue can be in a variety of areas:

Athlete's Foot (tinea pedis) - Over 10% of the U.S. population develops this problem. It is estimated that 75% of people will have athlete's foot at some time during their lifetimes. The most common form occurs between the toes, sometimes spreading to the sole of the foot. Between the toes, a person's skin becomes white, moist, and easily rubbed off. The tops of the toes may be red, dry, and flaky. Intense itching and burning are very common. Athlete's foot usually occurs with hot, moist conditions, or if a person wears shoes constantly.

Jock Itch (tinea cruris) - The same conditions of heat, moisture (sweat) and poor air circulation leading to athlete's foot also cause fungus infections of the groin, or jock itch. There is usually intense itching and burning in the perineal area and redness, flaking and peeling on the inner thighs, pubic area, and scrotum.

Ringworm (tinea corpora) - This is caused by a microscopic fungus. The infected area spreads out slowly from its central starting point and creates a slightly raised, intensely red ring surrounding a less red, flaky, itchy area. Over time, the ring slowly enlarges. It can occur anywhere on the body and appear in multiple sites at once, so it's often confused with other kinds of skin issues.

Candidiasis - This brownish-red, itchy discoloration affects the underarms, corners of the mouth, rectal area, and beneath the breasts.

Tinea Versicolor - This fungus changes the color of the skin it infects; the patches may be lighter or darker than your normal surrounding skin. This spotted pattern and the fine scaly flakes at the margins make this fungal infection the easiest to identify; itching and irritation are mild.

MANAGEMENT OF FUNGAL INFECTIONS
Personal Hygiene
- Use anti-perspirants and talcum powder to keep high-risk areas dry
  o Avoid use of baby powders or perfume scented powders
- If a person is susceptible to athlete's foot, encourage use an anti-fungal powders
- When in high heat and humid climates, keep the person's clothing loose and light; avoid knits and less breathable synthetic materials

Avoidance
- Use a clean towel/washcloth daily and do not share towels or clothes.
- Have the person wear thong sandals or other footwear in public locker rooms, pools, and showers
- The person should always wear a thick T-shirt or sweatshirt and long shorts or sweat pants while sharing exercise equipment
- Wipe off vinyl surfaces with a dry towel before using exercise equipment

Athlete's Foot – Tolnaftate is the only over the counter medicine approved for both prevention and treatment of athlete's foot. Be patient, though. It may take a more than a month of daily treatment for it to completely clear the problem. Consider preventive use if the condition recurs.

Tinea Versicolor – Selenium sulfide shampoo is often used and is recognized by dermatologists as an effective over the counter remedy. Since this condition often affects large areas of the trunk, applying this shampoo once a day for five minutes, then washing it off may be a lot easier and cheaper than using a whole tube of anti-fungal cream twice daily. Tinea versicolor also may recur and this shampoo can prevent that if it used once a week after the initial 2-4 week treatment cycle.

Candidiasis, Ringworm, and Jock Itch – Miconazole or clotrimazole are quickly effective (1-2 weeks) for each one of these conditions, and come in cream, lotion, or spray. Avoid alcohol-based products, since they can sting chafed and delicate skin. (Merck Manual for Geriatrics, 2010; Mayo Clinic, 2010; eMedicineNet.com, 2010; GNRS, 2007; Touhy & Jett, 2010)

Keratosis (also known as a solar keratosis), is a small, rough spot occurring on skin that has been chronically exposed to the sun. They generally measure in size between 2-6 millimeters in diameter (between the size of a pencil point and that of an eraser). They may be reddish in color, with a rough texture, and often have a white or yellowish scale on top. They often occur against a background of sun damage, including sallowness, wrinkles, and superficial blood vessels. Any elder who develops any lesion should be evaluated by a healthcare professional.

Cellulitis is a common skin infection caused by bacteria. Symptoms include fever with signs of infection: chills, shaking, fatigue, general ill feeling (malaise), possible muscle aches, pains (myalgias), redness and warm skin with possible sweating. Other symptoms include pain or tenderness in the area with the rash or sore; skin redness or inflammation that increases in size as the infection spreads; and skin soreness with a rash (macule). These come on suddenly, grow quickly in the first 24 hours, and usually exhibit sharp borders, tight, glossy, "stretched" appearance of the skin, and warmth over the area of redness. There may be swollen lymph nodes (lymphadenopathy). Other symptoms that can occur with this disease: hair loss at the site of infection; joint stiffness caused by swelling of the tissue over the joint; and fever, as well as nausea and vomiting if the infections gets into a person's system. Tests that may be necessary are: Culture & Sensitivity tests of wound drainage, Blood culture, and Complete blood count (CBC).

MANAGEMENT includes antibiotic ointment if the skin infection is localized. If the infection is associated with systemic symptoms or is fast progressing – consultation by a healthcare professional may be warranted to obtain appropriate treatment.

Lower Leg Ulcers are wounds or open sores on the lower extremity that keep returning or will not heal. The ulcer(s) may or may not be painful. The individual generally has a swollen leg and may feel burning or itching and the skin may exhibit a rash, redness, brown discoloration or dry, scaly appearance. Ulcers are typically defined by such characteristics as the appearance of the ulcer, the ulcer location, and the way the borders and surrounding skin of the ulcer look.

The three most common types of leg and foot ulcers include:
- Venous (stasis) ulcers
- Arterial (ischemic) ulcers
- Neurotrophic (diabetic) ulcers

Causes of Lower Extremity Ulcers
- Poor circulation, often caused by arteriosclerosis
- Venous insufficiency (a failure of the valves in the veins of the leg that causes congestion and slowing of blood circulation in the veins)
- Other disorders of clotting and circulation
- Diabetes
- Renal (kidney) failure
- Hypertension
- Lymphedema (a buildup of fluid that causes swelling in the legs or feet)
- Inflammatory diseases including vasculitis, lupus, scleroderma or other rheumatological conditions
- Other medical conditions such as high cholesterol, heart disease, high blood pressure, sickle cell anemia, bowel disorders
- Presently smoking or a history of smoking
- Pressure caused by lying in one position for too long
- Genetics (ulcers may be hereditary)
- A malignancy (tumor or cancerous mass)
- Infections
- Certain medications   (Mayo Clinic, 2010; MedicineNet.com, 2010)

Venous ulcers are often located below the knee and are primarily found on the inner part of the leg, just above the ankle. Often the individual has swelling or edema of the legs and feet. The base of a venous ulcer is usually red and may also be covered with yellow fibrous tissue. There may be drainage at the site with yellow or green discharge if the ulcer is infected. The borders of a venous ulcer are usually irregularly shaped and the surrounding skin is often discolored and swollen – possibly boggy (soft and fluid-filled surrounding the ulcer). The area may feel warm or hot. The surrounding skin may appear shiny and tight, depending on the amount of edema (swelling). Venous stasis ulcers are common in patients who have a history of leg swelling, varicose veins, or a history of blood clots in either the superficial or the deep veins of the legs. Ulcers can affect one leg or both legs. Venous ulcers affect a significant number of elders and are the most common ulcers of all the ulcers affecting the lower extremities.

Arterial ulcers are usually located on an elder's feet and often occur on the heels, tips of toes, between the toes where the toes rub against one another or anywhere the bones may protrude and rub against bed sheets, socks or shoes. They also occur commonly in the nail bed if the toenail cuts into the skin or if there has been recent aggressive toe nail trimming or an ingrown toenail removed. The base of an arterial ulcer usually does not bleed. It may have a yellow, brown, grey, or black color. The borders and surrounding skin usually appear sunken in. If irritation or infection is present, there may or may not be swelling and redness around the ulcer base. There may also be redness on the entire foot when the leg is dangled; this redness often turns to a pale white/yellow color when the leg is elevated. Arterial ulcers are often very painful, especially at night. (Mayo Clinic, 2010; eMedicineNet.com, 2010; GNRS, 2007; Touhy & Jett, 2010)

Diabetic ulcers are also referred to as neurotrophic ulcers and are usually located at increased pressure points on the bottom of the feet. These ulcers are related to trauma, which can occur anywhere on the foot. They occur primarily in people with diabetes, although they can affect anyone who has an impaired sensation of the feet (peripheral neuropathy). The base of the ulcer is variable is size and shape, depending on the elder's circulation. It may appear pink/red or brown/black. The borders of the ulcer may be punched out, while the surrounding skin is often calloused. But the borders may also be edematous with bogginess/softness of the surrounding skin. Neuropathy and peripheral artery disease often occur concurrently in elders who have diabetes. Nerve damage (neuropathy) in the feet can result in a loss of foot sensation and changes in the sweat-producing glands, increasing the risk of being unaware of foot calluses or cracks, injury or risk of infection. Symptoms of neuropathy include tingling, numbness, burning sensation or pain.

PREVENTION IS THE KEY – Individuals with diabetes need to inspect their feet and their shoes daily and wear appropriate footwear. Elders with diabetes should never walk barefoot (Mayo Clinic, 2010; eMedicineNet.com, 2010; GNRS, 2007; Touhy & Jett, 2010).

PREVENTION FOR ELDERS AT RISK FOR DEVELOPING PRESSURE ULCERS
- Have decreased mobility or are bed-bound
- Are incontinent of urine and/or feces
- Are cognitively impaired
- Have decreased sensations due to neuropathy or dementia

For 'at risk' elders, prevention begins with:
- Avoiding friction and shear trauma to skin regions
- Avoiding maceration from moisture
- Nutrition
  - Encourage a balanced diet & Vitamin C & Zinc daily, if an ulcer is present
- Incontinence
  - Keep the skin clean and dry
  - Air at night (open pads)
- Avoid lifestyle behaviors that impair wound healing
  - Smoking
  - Scratching
  - Immobility
- Addressing nutrition and mobility
  - Frequent repositioning – at least every 1 to 2 hours and more often if necessary
  - If sitting in a chair – shift weight every 15 minutes if possible

Inspect skin daily for high-risk elders
Skin and deep-tissue injury can occur in as little as two hours. Thus, high-risk elders may need daily skin examination.
- Identify and manage underlying medical risk factors, including disease states, nutritional compromise, skin disorders, and drugs that affect skin, such as corticosteroids
- Identify and treat modifiable causes of decreased alertness, incontinence, and immobility
- Identify changes that increase risk, such as weight loss or progression of dementia.
- Clarify overall condition, prognosis, and realistic goals

Managing Pressure Ulcers/Treatment

There are general guidelines that are currently accepted principles of treatment, which include the following components:

- Relieve pressure
- Remove (also referred to as Debridement) necrotic (dead) tissue
- Treat infection
- Keep the wound moist to promote healing
- Protect surrounding skin
- Manage the elder's overall condition
- Track wound-healing progress accurately

The most common sites of a pressure ulcer are Boney Prominences including:

- Buttocks/Sacrum
- Hips
- Heels
- Ankles/Feet
- Knees
- Elbows
- Wrists
- Shoulders
- Head
- Spine
- Ears

MANAGING LOWER EXTREMITY ULCERS

- Antibiotics, if an infection is present
- Blood thinning: Anti-platelet or anti-clotting medications to prevent a blood clot
- Topical wound care therapies
- Compression garments
- Prosthetics or orthotics, available to restore or enhance normal lifestyle function
- Keep the wound clean and dry
- Change the dressing as directed
- Have the person take prescribed medications as directed
- Drink plenty of fluids
- Follow a healthy diet, as recommended, including eating plenty of fruits and vegetables
- Exercise regularly, as directed by a physician
- Wear appropriate shoes
- Wear compression wraps, if appropriate, as directed

Venous stasis ulcers
- Moist to moist dressings: Wet-to-dry dressing (saline)
- Hydrogels/hydrocolloids: a debriding agent (such as Hydrogel) daily to assist in removal of necrotic (dead) tissue until any necrotic tissue or slough is resolved; cover with a moist dressing
- If drainage is present (Alginate dressings: calcium alginate daily and cover with dressing)
- Collagen wound dressings
- Antimicrobial dressings (silver alginate)
- Composite dressings
- Synthetic skin substitutes for large areas that will not heal
- Prevent pressure
- Prevent new ulcers

Arterial Insufficiency ulcers
- Position the extremity to promote circulation
- Provide adequate protection of the surface of the skin
- Apply a west Saline dressing to promote healing
- Consider antibiotic ointment daily if not healing
- Prevent new ulcers
- Remove contact irritation to the existing ulcer
- Monitor for signs and symptoms of infection that may involve the soft tissues or bone

(Mayo Clinic, 2010; eMedicineNet.com, 2010; GNRS, 2007; Touhy & Jett, 2010)

STAGING and MANAGING A PRESSURE ULCER

Staging a pressure ulcer is the key to determining how to treat the ulcer to promote healing. Note certain characteristics of an ulcer: the location, size (in centimeters, if possible), shape, appearance of the edges or outline, the color of the ulcer tissue and any surrounding skin, whether or not drainage if present, and if there is any odor present.

Stage 1 Ulcer: intact skin with non-blanchable redness of a localized area, usually occurs over a bony prominence, may be darkly pigmented skin that does not have visible blanching, and the color of the area may differ from surrounding skin. It may also be softer or boggy when you feel the area. It will usually hurt when you press on it, if the person can feel pain at the site.

Managing a Stage 1 Ulcer: prevent further skin damage and maintain intact skin; assess skin to assure healing and that the ulcer has not worsened; determine and remove the cause (such a pressure or incontinence) and implement.

Prevention Protocol: Provide repositioning of an immobile elder at least every 2 hours, frequent skin inspection, a balanced diet, moisture (incontinence) management, and evaluate progress.

Location: If on the heels, ankles, shoulders, elbows, wrists, spine, or head region: apply lubricating agent such as Proderm Spray daily & pad to prevent further pressure.

If on the Sacrum, coccyx, or hips: Assess vascular status condition for tolerance of film dressing – if good vascularization (blood supply) – apply a protective barrier such as Tegaderm or Duoderm dressing or apply thin Hydrocolloid dressing. If there is not good vascularization – consider a protective barrier cream (such as Laniseptic Cream, Baza cream, Boudreaux's Butt Paste, etc.) daily and as needed.

Stage 2 Ulcer has partial thickness loss of dermis – it may be a shallow open ulcer with a red pink wound bed, without slough. It may also present with intact skin (no break in the skin) or an open/ruptured serum-filled blister. They are usually superficial and may be persistent, such as an abrasion, blister, or shallow crater, with or without drainage.

Management includes maintaining a moist wound bed and avoiding maceration. Determine and remove the cause of the pressure and attempt to restore skin integrity and prevent further tissue damage. If the wound bed appears wet, treatment should be aimed at drying the ulcer: Clean with normal saline and fill with a cream/gel (such as calcium alginate) to draw out the moisture/drainage and apply dressing daily. *If the wound bed appears infected (colored drainage, an odor, or a non-healing ulcer) – consider a cream with antimicrobial properties such as silver alginate. If the wound bed appears dry, treatment should be aimed at moistening the ulcer: clean with normal saline and apply a moisture retentive dressing (such as a hydrocolloid, hydroactive dressing, thin foam, hydrogel sheet) daily. Consider adding Vitamin C 500 mg, Zinc 50 mg and Multivitamin daily to promote wound healing. And consider evaluation with specialists such as a dietitian, wound specialist, occupational therapist, and/or physiotherapist/physical therapist.

Stage 3 Ulcer is a full thickness tissue loss over an area. There may be subcutaneous fat visible in the wound bed, but bone, tendon, and/or muscle are not exposed. There may be slough present (loose skin that appears very fragile or necrotic), but this tissue does not obscure the depth of tissue loss. There may be undermining and tunneling of the ulcer to surrounding areas. The key to differentiating a stage 3 from a stage 4 ulcer is that there is no visible bone/tendon and the bone/tendon is not directly palpable.

Stage 4 Ulcer has full thickness skin loss with extensive destruction, tissue necrosis (dead tissue), or damage to muscle, bone, or supporting structures (such as the tendon, joint capsule). The stage 4 ulcer may tunnel or develop openings to other areas (tracks).

Managing Stage 3 & Stage 4 Ulcers: Prevent further tissue injury. Remove or debride non-viable tissue, absorb heavy drainage, fill wound dead space (open cavity of the wound) to promote healing from base of wound, and prevent infection. If there is necrotic tissue (black, dark brown, or maroon tissue– immediate evaluation by a healthcare provider is necessary). Consider adding Vitamin C 500 mg, Zinc 50 mg and Multivitamin daily to promote wound healing. And consider evaluation by specialists such as a dietitian, wound specialist, occupational therapist, and/or physiotherapist/physical therapist.

Implement Prevention Protocol PLUS: Rehydrate the area using hydrogel cream, foam, or dressing. Obtain an evaluation from a wound care specialist for management.

An Unstageable Ulcer or Deep Tissue Injury is difficult to assess and manage because the full extent of the ulcer is not apparent. There may be purple or maroon discoloration in a localized area of intact skin; or it may be a blood-filled blister due to damage of underlying soft tissue from pressure and/or shear; or the area may be preceded by tissue, as compared to adjacent tissue. It will usually be painful; it may be firm, soft or mushy or boggy to touch; and it may feel warmer or cooler than surrounding skin. Management is aimed at preventing further tissue injury; treating any infection which may be present; removing or eliminating necrotic (dead) tissue. If drainage is present, use an absorbent cream or gel to remove any heavy exudate and fill open space, in order to promote would healing. The goal of pressure ulcer care is to stage all wounds accurately, develop an appropriate plan of care, reassess the area often, and change management accordingly.

(Berlowitz & Wilking, 1989; Brandeis, Morris, Nash, & Lipsitz, 1990; Reed, 1981; Salcido & Popescu, 2009; SCHIMA, 2010)

KEY THINGS TO REMEMBER IN ULCER MANAGEMENT
- Wash hands thoroughly before and after treating the wound
- Wear gloves, so both the elder and the caregiver are protected from germs
- Gather together all of the materials needed for a dressing change before getting started
- When doing a sterile dressing change, set up the sterile field first; keep the sterile supplies away from the clean supplies
- Discard old dressing materials carefully; place the soiled wound dressings in a plastic bag, tie and dispose of it according to the community regulations
- Store solutions and dressing products carefully, according to the specific recommendations from a healthcare professional; ask if refrigeration of any treatment products is necessary to assist in prolonging the product shelf life
- Discard used solutions and dressing products according to the recommendations from a healthcare professional; ask about reusing certain products
- If any dressing products become wet or dirty, discard the entire package
- Use each dressing only once

(AHCPR, 1994)

Herpes Zoster or **Shingles** is a painful, blistering skin rash due to the varicella-zoster virus, the same virus that causes chickenpox. The person is exposed to the virus earlier in their lifetime and the virus remains inactive (becomes dormant) in certain nerves in the body. Shingles occur after the virus becomes active again in these nerves years later, especially when an elder is stressed due to illness, surgery, physical stress, or emotional stress.

Risk Factors increase a person's chances of developing the symptoms of shingles – if the person is over the age of 60, had chickenpox before age 1, or if their immune system is weakened by medications or disease. The first symptom is usually pain on one side of the body or face; it may be experienced as tingling, hurting, or burning. It may be severe and is usually present before any rash appears. Symptoms (such red patches on the skin, followed by small blisters) occur in most people. The blisters may be fluid filled and break open, forming smaller ulcers that begin to dry and form crusts. The crusts fall off in 2 to 3 weeks. Scarring is usually rare. The rash typically involves a narrow area from the spine around to the front of the belly area or chest. Or the rash may involve face, eyes, mouth, and ears. Additional symptoms may include: abdominal pain, chills, difficulty moving some of the muscles in the face, drooping eyelid (ptosis), fever and chills, general ill-feeling, genital lesions, headache, hearing loss, joint pain, loss of eye motion, swollen glands (lymph nodes), taste problems, and/or vision problems.

Management in elders is aimed at prevention and symptoms management, as well as decreasing the number of outbreaks and the severity of an outbreak. There is a Shingles Vaccination, which is a one-time shot that can be given even if a person has a history of Shingles – it will decrease the severity of the outbreaks. Shingles symptoms usually disappear spontaneously. Treatment is usually aimed relieving the associated pain and preventing infection of any open skin areas. Antiviral Agents may help reduce pain and complications and shorten the course of the disease: acyclovir (Zovirax) twice a day for 5-7 days. Alternative agents: famciclovir (Famvir) and valacyclovir (Valtrex). The medications should be started within 24 hours of feeling pain or burning, and preferably before the blisters appear. The drugs are usually given in pill form, in doses many times greater than those recommended for herpes simplex or genital herpes. Some people may need to receive the medicine through a vein (by IV). Other medications used to manage the symptoms include strong anti-inflammatory medicines called corticosteroids, such as prednisone, which may be used to reduce swelling and the risk of continued pain. These drugs do not work in all elders and may cause anxiety and agitation in certain elders. Other medicines may include: antihistamines to reduce itching (taken by mouth or applied to the skin), pain medicines, and Zostrix, a cream containing capsaicin (an extract of pepper) to prevent postherpetic neuralgia. Management also includes applying cool wet compresses to reduce pain; cool, soothing baths and lotions, such as colloidal oatmeal bath, starch baths, or calamine lotion to relieve itching and discomfort; and resting in bed if the person is running a fever. The skin should be kept clean, and only clean dressings and clothing should be used – discard any articles contaminated with the drainage. All nondisposable items should be washed in boiling water or otherwise disinfected before reuse. The individual may need to be isolated while lesions are oozing to prevent infection of others.

(Mayo Clinic, 2010; eMedicineNet.com, 2010; GNRS, 2007; Touhy & Jett, 2010)

Chapter 10 References

AHCPR. (1994). Treating pressure sores. Consumer Version Clinical Practice Guideline Number 15. Agency for Health Care Policy and Research (AHCPR), U.S. Department of Health and Human Services.

Berlowitz, D.R., Wilking, S.V. (1989) Risk factors for pressure sores. A comparison of cross-sectional and cohort-derived data. *Journal of American Geriatrics Society*; 37(11):1043-50.

Brandeis, G.H., Morris, J.N., Nash, D.J., Lipsitz, L.A. (1990) The epidemiology and natural history of pressure ulcers in elderly nursing home residents. *JAMA*; 264(22):2905-9

eMedicine.Net (2010) Skin Anatomy. Retrieved December 30, 2010, from http://emedicine.medscape.com/article/1294744-overview

eMedicine.Net (2010) Life threatening skin lesions. Retrieved December 30, 2010, from http://www.emedicinehealth.com/life-threatening_skin_rashes/article_em.htm

GNRS (2007). Dermatological diseases and disorders. AGS: New York.

Hogan, D. (2010). Corns. Retrieved September 3, 2010, from http://emedicine.medscape.com/article/1089807-overview

Mayo Clinic (2010). Skin cancer. Retrieved December 30, 2010, from http://www.mayoclinic.com/health/skin-cancer/DS00190

Mayo Clinic (2010). Skin care. Retrieved December 30, 2010, from http://www.mayoclinic.com/health/skin-care/SN00003

Merck Manual for Geriatrics Online (2010). Common Skin Disorders. Retrieved December 30, 2010, from http://www.merckmanuals.com/professional/sec23.html

Reed, J.W. (1981) Pressure ulcers in the elderly: prevention and treatment utilizing the team approach. *Maryland State Medical Journal.* 30(11):45-50.

Salcido, R. & Popescu, A. (2009). Pressure Ulcers and Wound Care-Updated 2006. Retrieved January 16, 2009, from http://www.emedicine.medscape.com

SCHIMA State Coding Roundtable November 7, 2008. Retrieved January 16, 2009, from http://www.npuap.org; http://www.wocn.org; http://www.nursingquality.org; http://www.ihi.org; and http://www.5millionlives.premierinc.com

Touhy & Jett (2010). Ebersole and Hess' Gerontological Nursing and Healthy Aging. 3rd ed. Mosby-Elsevier: Missouri; 163-178.

Treating pressure sores. (1994). Consumer Version Clinical Practice Guideline Number 15. Agency for Health Care Policy and Research (AHCPR), U.S. Department of Health and Human Services.

Summary

This Chapter presents a summary of geriatric care, including caution in geriatric dosing, laboratory monitoring, polypharmacy (multiple medication usage, inappropriate medications used in elders, and drug interactions), and hints to optimize health in elders.

There are a few additional issues to consider in the health of older individuals. Many elders use a significant number of medications and – although many are necessary – all medications have side effects, interact with other medications, and must be used judiciously in order to optimize health and minimize problems. Many elders are taking multiple medications; it is estimated that a significant number of elders take 5 or more medications on a daily basis. There is potentially inappropriate and/or excessive use of both prescription medications and over-the-counter medications and herbal supplements by elders.

Problems are often caused by or can be increased by taking

- Medication dosages that are too high
- Medications that are incorrectly prescribed or filled (not taken as prescribed)
- Medications that interact with or duplicate the actions of other medications
- Over-the-counter, non-prescription medications that cause health problems or interact with prescription medications
- Herbal supplements/remedies that that cause health problems or interact with prescription medications

Summary

Polypharmacy is the use of more than 5 medications on a daily basis; it can result in adverse drug events, which may complicate therapy, increase the cost, and present a challenge for prescribers. Unfortunately, the symptoms caused by polypharmacy can be confused with the normal aging process; these include:

- Tiredness, sleepiness, or decreased alertness
- Constipation, diarrhea, or incontinence
- Loss of appetite
- Confusion
- Falls
- Depression or lack of interest in one's usual activities
- Weakness
- Tremors
- Visual or auditory hallucinations
- Anxiety or excitability
- Dizziness
- Decreased sexual behavior

The issue of inappropriate prescribing in the geriatric population is an extremely important one, especially since this population consumes a large percentage of all prescription medications (over 25%), though it forms only about 12% of the total United States population (but continues to grow) (Balogun et al, 2005). Polypharmacy is especially worrisome in the elderly because of an increased risk for adverse drug reactions, multiple co-morbid disease processes, and multiple medication use leading to medication interactions; polypharmacy has also been linked to an increased risk of hospitalization and death in elders.

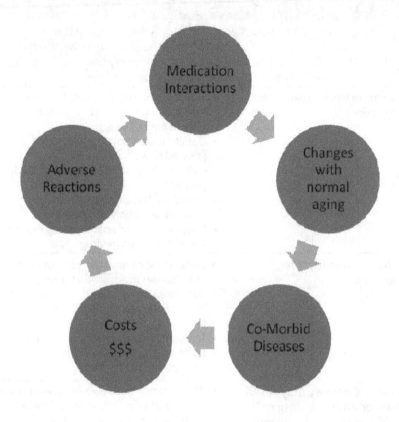

Figure 11-1. *Polypharmacy in Elders*

Table 11-1. *Factors to Consider in Medication Use in Elders*	
Medications can interact with one another and cause potential problems. There are certain medications that are more worrisome than others. Below are some of the most commonly seen medication interaction problems in Nursing Home residents	
Gastrointestinal absorption or function	• Slowing of gastrointestinal transit time may prolong the effects of continuous release enteral drugs • Opioid-related bowel dysmotility (slowed bowel motility and constipation) may be enhanced in older patients • Disorders that alter gastric pH may reduce absorption of some drugs • Surgically altered anatomy may reduce absorption of some drugs
Topical or Transdermal absorption	• Under most circumstances, there are few changes in absorption through the skin based on age, but this may relate more to different medications or patch technology used • Temperature and other specific patch technology characteristics may affect absorption
Aging and obesity may result in longer effective drug half-life (*drugs stay in the system longer and the level may be increased in the blood*)	• Distribution – Increased fat to lean body weight ratio may increase volume of distribution for fat soluble drugs • Oxidation is variable and may decrease, resulting in prolonged drug half-life
Liver metabolism (*how medications are metabolized*)	• Conjugation is usually preserved • First-pass effect is usually unchanged • Genetic enzyme polymorphisms may affect some cytochrome enzymes • Cirrhosis, hepatitis, tumors may disrupt oxidation but not usually conjugation

(CONTINUED)

Table 11-1. *Factors to Consider in Medication Use in Elders (CONTINUED)*

Renal excretion *(how medications are filtered out of the body)*	• Glomerular filtration rate decreases with advancing age in many patients, which results in decreased excretion • Chronic kidney disease may predispose the person further to renal toxicity
Active Metabolites	• Reduced renal clearance will prolong the effects of metabolites • Renal disease – Increase in half-life
Anticholinergic side effects	• Certain medications have anticholinergic effects, which lead to an increased chance an elder will develop confusion, constipation, incontinence, movement disorders, falls, and agitation • Certain medications are enhanced by neurological disease processes, including Alzheimer's disease and many of the dementias

AGS (2010)

WAYS TO DECREASE POLYPHARMACY IN ELDERS

1. Annually review all medications for potentially inappropriate medications and reduction of unnecessary medications
2. Prioritize Necessary vs. Optional medications
3. Limit or discontinue use of agents used on an 'as needed' basis, especially if they are not being used very often
4. Document and determine reason why taking a medication (indication) for every medication – Drugs with no indications should be stopped
5. Avoid treating adverse reactions/side effects with more drugs
   a. For example – managing edema caused by a calcium channel blocker with a diuretic such a furosemide
6. Judicious use of medications which can cause problems in elders:
   a. Psychotropic agents: benzodiazepines
   b. Anti-hypertensive agents
   c. Diuretics
   d. Digoxin
   e. NSAIDS
   f. Corticosteroids
   g. Warfarin
   h. Theophylline
7. Geriatric tips for Prescribing in Elders:

Summary

a. Prefer single dose regimens (once a day dosing)
b. Limit the use of 'as needed' medications
c. Consider all new medications as a therapeutic trial – see if the medication results in benefits with no problems due to the medication
d. Discontinue a medication if it is ineffective or has intolerable adverse side effects
e. Certain medications should be weaned off; weanable medications:
   i. Antipsychotics should receive a trail dose reduction every 6 months until medication is discontinued – NOTE: if the elder has recurrence of problems or psychotic behaviors, increase the antipsychotic back to the original dose and wait 3 months then re-attempt dose reduction. If the symptoms recur and there have been two attempts to wean/stop the medication, then the medication is necessary; document these findings – no further dose reductions may be necessary; the benefits outweigh the risks of use
   ii. Appetite stimulants should be reduced and discontinued – monitor weight weekly for 4 weeks - if no change in weight, the medication was not helping
   iii. Alzheimer's agents in advanced dementia – if an elder is unable to feed self, turn self, or speak in more than a 3-word sentence, anticholinesterase inhibitors such as Aricept or Exelon may not be helping – try a discontinuance of the medication. Monitor the elder and, if necessary, restart the medication within 4 weeks. There may be a need to restart if psychiatric problems occur, such as decreasing intake, or if behavioral problems occur, such as crying, scratching self, grimacing more often, etc.
f. Attempt to prescribe a medication that will treat more than one existing problem-Examples:
   i. Calcium channel blocker or beta blocker to treat both hypertension and angina pectoris
   ii. ACE-inhibitor to treat hypertension, heart failure, and/or renal protection in diabetics
   iii. Alpha-blocker to treat hypertension and prostatism
   iv. Cymbalta to treat depression and peripheral neuropathy or fibromyalgia

To review Beer's criteria for medications which are potentially inappropriate for use in elders, visit http://www.dcri.duke.edu/ccge/curtis/beers.html

DRUG INTERACTIONS

Elders are at an increased risk of adverse effects with certain drugs. The increased risk may be due to age-related changes in pharmacokinetics or pharmacodynamics. Risk of an adverse effect increases substantially when multiple drugs are used. Aging changes combined with the presence of multiple diseases such as hypertension and diabetes, makes an older person at increased rick for complications from medications as well as side effects of medications. (Merck Manual for Geriatrics, 2010).

There are certain drugs that interact with other medications which can cause major problems in elders.

Table 11-2. TOP 10 Dangerous Drug Interactions in Elders		

Warfarin (Coumadin) AND...	**NSAIDS**
	• Aleve
	• Anaprox
	• Ansaid
	• Feldene
	• Lodine
	• Ibuprofen
	• Ketoprofen
	• Mobic
	• Naprelan
	• Indomethacin
	• Orudis
	• Relafen
	• Volteran
		Increases effects of Coumadin *Potential GI bleed*
		• Alternative agents to use:
		  *For Fever or pain:
		  Use Acetaminophen
		  (no more than 2g/day)
		• For anti-inflammatory agent:
		  Use COX-2 inhibitor therapy

Warfarin (Coumadin) AND...	*Sulfanamides* • Bactrim • Septra • Triam/ Sulfamethoxazole	*Increases effects of Coumadin* *Potential GI bleed* • Decrease Coumadin dose while on antibiotic therapy (possibly decrease to every other day • Check PT with INR while on antibiotic therapy

(CONTINUED)

Warfarin (Coumadin) AND...	**Macrolides** • Azithromycin • Biaxin • Clarithromycin • Erythromycin • Pediazole	**Increases effects of Coumadin Potential GI bleed** • Decrease Coumadin dose while on antibiotic therapy (possibly decrease to every other day) • Check PT with INR while on antibiotic therapy
Warfarin (Coumadin) AND...	**Fluoroquinolones** • Avelox • Floxin • Levaquin • Ciprofloxin	**Increases effects of Coumadin Potential GI bleed** • Decrease Coumadin dose while on antibiotic therapy (possibly decrease to every other day) • Check PT with INR while on antibiotic therapy
Warfarin (Coumadin) AND...	**Phenytoin** • Dilantin • Phenytek	**Increases effects of Coumadin Consider** • Obtain baseline phenytoin levels
Ace Inhibitors (Accupril, Altace, Captopril, Capoten, Lisinopril, Mavik, Prinivil, Quinopril, Univasc, Vasotec, Zestril) AND...	**Potassium Supplements** • KLor • KTab • KDur • Koon	**Potential increased potassium levels** • Consider obtaining baseline Potassium level and within one week after initiating therapy • Consider EKG monitoring
Ace Inhibitors (Accupril, Altace, Captopril, Capoten, Lisinopril, Mavik, Prinivil, Quinopril, Univasc, Vasotec, Zestril) AND...	**Spironolactone** • Aldactone	**Potential increased potassium levels** • Consider obtaining baseline Potassium level and within one week after initiating therapy • Consider EKG monitoring

(CONTINUED)

Table 11-2. TOP 10 Dangerous Drug Interactions in Elders (CONTINUED)

Digoxin (Lanoxin) AND...	**Amiodarone** • Cardarone • Pacerone	**Potential Digoxin toxicity** • Consider obtaining digoxin level prior to initiating Amiodarone and decrease digoxin dose by ½ then check Digoxin level weekly for several weeks
Digoxin (Lanoxin) AND...	**Verapamil** • Calan • Covera • Isoptin • Verelan	**Potential Digoxin toxicity** • synergistic effect slowing impulse conduction & muscle contractility • bradycardia, & possible heart block * Consider monitoring EKG, S/S Digoxin toxicity – abdominal pain, anorexia, changes in mentation, blurred vision, bradycardia, delirium, depression, diarrhea, halos around lights, nausea, neuralgia, nightmares, photophobia, vertigo, vomiting, weakness
Theophylline (Aminophylline, Slo-Bid, Theo-Dur, Theolair) AND...	**Fluoroquinolones** • Avelox • Cipro • Floxin • Levaquin • Norfloxacin • Tequin	**Potential theophylline toxicity** *(reduces theophylline clearance by 30 to 84%)* • Consider obtaining theophylline level baseline and after initiating therapy

Problems encountered when an elder is hospitalized
(Iatrogenic problems)

Aggressive care, as well as hospitalizations of an older person, often occur unexpectedly and are commonly due to a change in condition of an older person. An acute change in condition is a sudden, clinically-important deviation from the resident's physical, cognitive, behavioral, or functional status which could cause significant complications or death (Advancing Excellence, 2008). There are steps to monitor for and predict potential problems that could occur in elders with certain diagnoses:

1. identify all of an elder's medical conditions and match disease states with potential problems
2. identify elders at risk for poor outcomes
3. identify interventions that may reduce potential problems
4. report changes in condition promptly to the prescribing healthcare provider
5. assess and treat according to evidenced-based practice protocols
6. re-assess to assure improvement of an elder's condition.

There are acute changes in condition that do necessitate hospitalization, including acute abdominal pain of moderate to severe intensity with intractable vomiting; chest pain that cannot be readily attributed to non-cardiac causes; falls with potential fracture; hypertensive crises – SBP>230 mmHg; upper active gastrointestinal bleed with hypotension & tachycardia; and respiratory distress that does not respond to oxygen, nebulizer treatments, or suctioning (Advancing Excellence, 2008). Common diagnoses associated with acute hospitalizations (CMS, 2008):

- Respiratory Symptoms (Respiratory Distress, Pneumonia, Bronchitis, etc.)
- Urinary Tract Infections (UTI)
- Cerebrovascular Accidents (CVA)
- Cardiovascular Changes
- Falls
- Gastrointestinal Bleeding

Table 11-3. COMMON HEALTH PROBLEMS AND THEIR COMMON COMPLICATIONS	
Condition/Diagnosis	**Potential Problem**
Chronic Obstructive Pulmonary Disease	*Acute Dyspnea* *Respiratory Infections*
Diabetes	*Fluid/electrolyte imbalance* *Hyperglycemia* *Hypoglycemia* *Urinary Tract Infections/Yeast Infections*
Hip Fracture	*Deep Vein Thrombosis* *Pulmonary Embolus*
Gastrointestinal Bleed	*Acute recurrence of bleed*
Acute Myocardial Infarction	*Deep Vein Thrombosis* *Pulmonary Embolism* *Dysrhythmia*
Atrial fibrillation with anticoagulation/medication changes	*Bleeding* *Cerebrovascular Accident/Stroke*
Congestive Heart Failure	*Acute Dyspnea* *Pulmonary Edema*
Neurogenic Bladder	*Urinary Tract Infection*
New Medication	*Falls* *Delirium* *Respiratory Depression*
Parkinson's Disease	*Aspiration* *Agitation* *Change in Mental Status* *Falls* *Dysphagia*
Stroke/Cerebrovascular Accident	*Recurrence of Stroke* *Acute bleed due to anticoagulation*

Beginning immediately upon admission to an acute care setting, such as a hospital, vulnerable, frail elders are at increased risk for many problems, including worsening functional status, delirium, falls, medication toxicity, nosocomial infections, malnutrition, dehydration, immobilization, and decubitus ulcer (CMS, 2009; Walsh & Bruza, 2007). Research suggests ways to diminish a high portion of acute hospital transfers from a Nursing Home by providing a higher acuity of care at the Nursing Home (Advancing Excellence, 2008).
Ways to raise the acuity of care in LTC

- More skilled staffing, including a higher ratio of Registered Nurses (RNs)
- Education for all staff with a geriatric emphasis
- Consistency of assignments so staff know the patients & the norm for each patient
- Reporting acute changes in condition promptly
- Availability of laboratory results within 3 hours
- Ability to initiate & maintain intravenous hydration
- Establishment of a Protocol System and/or better implementation of Protocols

(Advancing Excellence, 2008)

Studies have shown that there were certain characteristics that correlated to a higher number of acute hospitalizations from nursing homes (Advancing Excellence, 2008):

- Higher number of certified beds
- Higher % Medicaid patients
- Lower % of Caucasian residents
- Fewer advanced directives
- Substantial problems accessing Healthcare Providers (Medical directors, Physicians, Nurse Practitioners, & Physician Assistants)
- Common Diagnoses in Elders residing in LTC and Potential Complications

Educating Staff in Nursing Homes

The focus should be geared initially to educating staff, having nurses and all caregivers being more knowledgeable and understanding, as well as monitoring for complications that are common with specific diseases/disorders in the geriatric population, and communicating between healthcare providers using appropriate and descriptive language, treating promptly, and providing appropriate follow-up care. Studies indicate that when a Healthcare Provider, such as a Physician, Nurse Practitioner or Physician's Assistant, is able to provide on-site evaluation at least 2 to 3 days a week, hospitalizations can potentially be decreased by an average of 33% – that would save Medicare $1.4 billion annually (Advancing Excellence, 2008). The key to delivering optimal care in long term care (nursing home) is to know the residents, know what problems could occur, identify acute changes in condition, and treat promptly. Ideally, if caregivers are monitoring for potential problems, are able to identify the nature, severity, and causes of the problems related to each individual's diagnoses, and to accurately evaluate and promptly manage problems, unnecessary transfers to an acute hospital setting can be prevented. While hospitalization is necessary for certain conditions, such as hip fracture and stroke, transfer to a hospital can often be discretionary for other conditions, such as pneumonia and influenza (CMS, 2009). Avoidable hospitalizations in elders who reside in long term care (nursing home) could improve quality of life for these individuals by allowing care to be provided in their usual setting, decreasing the exposure of elders to potential hospital-acquired complications, and delivering care in a more cost-effective manner.

Promoting Health in Elders

The nature of illness in older adults is changing due to longer life spans as a result of public health measures & advances in medicine. Many older individuals are typically living longer than they did in previous generations, even in the presence of acute diseases. Chronic diseases are more common now, and diseases such as diabetes and heart disease are the major cause of illness, disability, and death in elders, accounting for 75% of all current deaths. The elderly population uses 80% of all health resources in the United States as of 2010. This is due to the fact that people live longer with disabling chronic conditions. On average, by age 75, older adults have between two to three chronic medical conditions. Some have ten or twelve conditions and many of these individuals with chronic illness have special health care needs, which involve greater care coordination and need for access to non-clinical support services. The main goal is to prevent disease, prevent acute illness, diminish the effects of chronic diseases, and promote health to have a healthier older person. This will also improve quality of life and decrease costs. Health promotion in the elderly population should be a multifaceted approach to care of the older adult with the goals of:

- problem identification
- health promotion
- maintenance of health
- maintenance of independence

Assessment should include all aspects of an older person's health:
- Physical
- Psychological
- Social

When developing a plan of care, take into consideration:

1. an elder's preferences and
2. the family's preferences
- Aggressiveness of care – acute hospitalization, outpatient/community-based care, or nursing home care
- Advanced directives – what measures are acceptable and what measures are not
- Goals for care
  - o health
  - o preventive medicine
  - o cure
  - o symptom relief
  - o palliative care – comfort measures with the understanding that a cure is not an expectation of care

Rapid Screening of an Older Adult
Assess Function
- Activities of daily living – ADLs
  - o bathing, dressing, transferring from bed to chair, toileting, grooming, feeding self
- Instrumental Activities of daily living – IADLs
  - o using the telephone, preparing meals, managing household finances, taking medications, doing laundry, doing housework, shopping, managing transportation

- Mobility
  - Walking from room to room
  - Climbing stairs
  - Walking outside
- Nutrition
- Vision
- Hearing
- Cognition
- Depression

Health Promotion *Consider common health maintenance/illness prevention activities for older adults:*

Immunizations
- Influenza – annually
- Pneumonia – every 5 years
- Tetanus – every 10 years
- Shingles – once in a lifetime

Screenings
- Eyes – annually
- Dental – annually
- Skin – annually for most elders; – monthly for those individuals at risk for (or with a history of) skin cancer

Breast Cancer
- Screening mammograms should be done every two years beginning at age 50 for women at average risk of breast cancer
- There is insufficient evidence that mammogram screening is effective for women age 75 and older, so it's not recommended for this age group (2010-U.S. Preventive Services Task Force (USPSTF); 2009 – American Cancer Society)

Cervical Cancer
Pap Smear
- Beginning at age 30, women who have had 3 normal Pap test results in a row may get screened every 2 to 3 years. Women older than 30 may also get screened every 3 years with either the conventional or liquid-based Pap test, plus the human papilloma virus (HPV) test
- Women 70 years of age or older who have had 3 or more normal Pap tests in a row and no abnormal Pap test results in the last 10 years may choose to stop having Pap tests
- Women who have had a total hysterectomy (removal of the uterus and cervix) may also choose to stop having Pap tests, unless the surgery was done as a treatment for cervical cancer or pre-cancer; women who have had a hysterectomy without removal of the cervix should continue to have Pap tests

Colorectal Cancer

Beginning at age 50, both men and women should follow one of these testing schedules:
- Tests that find polyps and cancer
- Flexible sigmoidoscopy every 5 years, or
- Colonoscopy every 10 years, or
- Double-contrast barium enema every 5 years, or
- CT colonography (virtual colonoscopy) every 5 years

Tests that primarily find colon cancer
- Yearly fecal occult blood test (gFOBT), or
- Yearly fecal immunochemical test (FIT) every year, or
- Stool DNA test (sDNA), interval uncertain

Prostate Cancer
- Screening tests are often part of a routine physical exam, especially in men over age 40
- Prostate-Specific Antigen (PSA) Test – A sample of blood is analyzed for PSA, a substance produced in the prostate gland that helps liquefy semen (a small amount of PSA always circulates in the blood); high PSA levels, or levels that rise over time, could indicate prostate inflammation, enlargement, or cancer
- Also recommend screening tests because of symptoms pointing to a prostate problem

Prostatitis in males
- Annual Prostate Specific Antigen (PSA) – a blood test for men up to age 50
- Annual PSA recommended if an individual has a life expectancy of greater than 10 years or after age 70, annual PSA is not recommended
- If PSA elevated – unless >10, recheck in 2 to 6 months & watch for doubling of PSA
- Digital Rectal Exam (DRE) annually up to age 70 – gently insert a gloved, lubricated finger into the patient's rectum and, by pressing against the rectal wall, can feel the back wall of the prostate gland
- About 70 percent of cancerous tumors develop near the outer portion of the prostate and can be detected through a DRE

CONCLUSION

A healthy lifestyle can lead to a healthy older person. Much of the illness, disability, and death associated with chronic disease is avoidable through prevention. Key measures to practicing a healthy lifestyle include:

- regular physical activity
- healthy eating
- avoiding tobacco use – or stopping use
- limiting sun exposure, and using sunscreen to prevent skin cancer
- early detection practices
- screening for breast, cervical, and colorectal cancers
- screening for hypertension, diabetes, and dyslipidemia
- annual eye examinations
- mental health screening, including screening for depression

There are many changes that occur normally in individuals as they age. It is important to understand normal aging changes in order to differentiate them from pathological conditions. While the effects of aging on cells, tissues and organs are a normal part of aging, the good news is that these changes usually appear over a long period of time, and exercise and good nutrition can play an important part in keeping the body healthy longer (O'Brien, 2009). Healthcare providers must understand these changes in order to communicate to patients what to expect and ways to promote healthy aging.

Chapter 11 References

Advancing Excellence in Nursing Home Care Campaign (2008). Retrieved May 13, 2009, from http://www.nhqualitycampaign.org/star_index.aspx?controls=nursing_homes

AGS (2010). Pharmacological Management of Persistent Pain in Older Persons: American Geriatrics Society Panel on the Pharmacological Management of Persistent Pain in Older Persons. Retrieved May 13, 2009, from http://www.americangeriatrics.org/health_care_professionals/clinical_practice/clinical_guidelines_recommendations/persistent_pain_executive_summary

American Cancer Society (2010). Guidelines for early detection of cancer. Retrieved June 15, 2010, from http://www.cancer.org/docroot/ped/content/ped_2_3x_acs_cancer_detection_guidelines_36.asp

Balogun, S., Preston, M., & Evans, J. (2005). Potentially Inappropriate Medications in Nursing Homes: Sources and Correlates. *The Internet Journal of Geriatrics and Gerontology*. 2 (2). Retrieved March 9. 2010, from http://www.ispub.com/ostia/index.php?xmlFilePath=journals/ijgg/vol2n2/nursing.xml

Center for Medicare Services (CMS). (2008). Certain interventions have the potential to reduce costly and risky hospitalizations of the frail elderly. US Department of Health and Human Services-AHRQ-April 2008. Retrieved May 13, 2009, from http://www.ahrq.gov/research/apr08/0408RA14.htm

HelpGuide.org (2009). Nursing Homes: Skilled Nursing Facilities. Retrieved May 29, 2009, from http://www.helpguide.org/elder/nursing_homes_skilled_nursing_facilities.htm

Merck Manual for Geriatrics. (2010). Adverse Drug Effects in the Elderly. Retrieved December 30, 2010, from http://www.merckmanuals.com/professional/sec20/ch306/ch306d.html

Peterson, E. (2010). Aging Gracefully: Reducing the Risks of Polypharmacy. Retrieved March 12, 2010, from http://healthlibrary.epnet.com/GetContent.aspx?token=7e9094f4-c284-4b3a-8f7c-867fd12b36ee&chunkiid=45329

Straub, B. (2008). Perspectives from CMS: Towards Continuous Improvement in the Future. Centers for Medicare & Medicaid Services (CMS) 2008 American Health Quality Association Annual Meeting. Retrieved May 13, 2009, from http://www.ahqa.org/pub/uploads/CMSPlenary_PerspectivesCMS.ppt

Walsh, K., & Bruza, J. (2007). Hospitalization of the Elderly. *Annals of Long Term Care*. 15 (11)

Definitions & Terms

Acute pain begins suddenly and can be sharp in quality; it serves as a warning of a problem such as a disease or a threat to the body

Ageism is a type of stereotyping – a belief about elders that views aging individuals as having an expectation to become senile, confused, demented

Alzheimer's disease: A pathological disorder of the brain that causes chemical changes in a person's brain, cognitive impairment, and eventual shrinkage of the brain; the person develops strange clumps of protein (plaques) and tangled fibers inside the nerve cells of his brain

Anomia: difficulty naming objects

Anosmia: a diminished sense of smell

Anxious Symptoms: Anxiety; Restlessness; Chronic complaints such as pain, constipation, insomnia, etc.; Muscle irritability; Irritability; Concentration problems; Headaches, backaches or digestive problems; Insomnia

Aphasia: Difficulty using and/or understanding language

Aspiration: An abnormal problem in which saliva, food, or fluid enters the lungs

Asymptomatic Bacteriuria: A condition characterized by a bacterial count in the urine absent of symptoms such as dysuria, urinary frequency, incontinence of recent onset, flank pain, fever, or other signs of infection

Auditory hallucination: Hearing sounds or people talking that are not real; some people who experience auditory hallucinations where the individual has conversations with people who are not really there, including deceased loved ones

Chronic pain: Pain lasting longer than one month or pain that continues despite the fact that the cause of pain has resolved or an injury has healed; also referred to as 'persistent pain'

Constipation: Difficult or infrequent passage of stool, hardness of stool, or a feeling of incomplete evacuation of the colon with defecation

Cystitis: The medical term for inflammation of the bladder

Deconditioning: Decreased activity tolerance in an older person

Delirium: a sudden severe confusion and rapid changes in mentation of a person – occurring over a few hours to a few days with markedly increased changes in level of consciousness, including confusion and agitation

Delusion: is a belief that is untrue, but the event is not out of context with a person's social and cultural background

Delusional misidentification: may result from a combined decline in visual function and recent memory problems: individuals may suspect that a family member is an impostor, believe that strangers are living in their home, or fail to recognize their own reflection in a mirror

Definitions & Terms

Dementia: Not a disease itself but a group of symptoms, caused by various diseases or conditions with symptoms that include changes in personality, mood, and behavior. It is the loss of mental functions such as thinking, memory, and reasoning which is severe enough to interfere with a person's ability to carry out the daily tasks of living

Depressed Symptoms: No interest or pleasure in things one used to enjoy, including sex; Feeling sad or numb; Crying easily or for no reason; Feeling slowed down; Feeling worthless or guilty; Change in appetite; unintended change in weight; Trouble recalling things, concentrating or making decisions; Problems sleeping, or wanting to sleep all of the time; Feeling tired all of the time; Thoughts about death or suicide

Disinhibition: A lack of social skills and restraint to adhere to social norms which can be manifested in several ways, including disregard for acceptable behaviors, poor risk assessment, and impulsivity; an individual suffering from dementia is less able to exercise normal control: to choose to inhibit some responses in the way most people would do each day for reasons of politeness, sensitivity, social appropriateness, or desire to keep our true feelings hidden from others

Durable Power of Attorney: A document which assigns another individual to make medical decisions and authorizes that person to make financial decisions; this allows another person to make decisions regarding healthcare and to sign medical consent forms (it also allows the person access to an individual's bank accounts and finances, gives authority to sell property, and make decisions regarding the elder's living environment) – a person authorizes this while he/she is legally capable of making decisions and the document is filed in a Court of Law in the county/state where the person resides

Durable Financial Power of Attorney: A document which authorizes another person to make only financial decisions; this allows another person access to bank accounts and finances and gives the person authority to sell property; a person authorizes this while he/she is legally capable of making decisions and the document filed in a Court of Law in the county/state where the person resides

Dyarthria: A problem where physically producing speech is difficult

Dystonia: A neurological movement disorder, in which sustained muscle contractions cause twisting and repetitive movements or abnormal postures

Dysuria: Burning sensations with urination

Expressive aphasia: An inability to verbalize what a person is thinking

Guardianship: A legal manner in which an individual who is unable to make decisions has another individual make decisions for him/her; if an individual is no longer competent to make decisions due to Alzheimer's disease or another disease process – if there is no Advanced Directive or Durable Power of Attorney in place, and if there is no relative who is available to make decisions for the individual – the courts will assign a Guardian to make medical and financial decisions for the person

Hallucination: A false sensory perception not related merely to distortions or misinterpretations; auditory hallucinations are hearing sounds or voices that are not real and visual hallucinations are seeing objects, colors, or visions that are not real

Hematuria: blood in the urine

Hyperphagia: disinhibition with social conventions to repress placing objects in a person's mouth; this can be expressed as behaviors like constantly eating, placing things in one's mouth, chewing constantly, or smacking lips frequently

Hypersexuality: disinhibition with social conventions to repress sexual urges; this can be expressed with behaviors such as being preoccupied with sexual demands or with fondling oneself or others

Hypersomnia: Excessive daytime sleepiness over a long period of time

Indigestion: a common cause of alteration in appetite for an elder, defined as discomfort in the upper abdomen such as bloating, belching and nausea

Insomnia: inability to fall asleep, night-time awakenings, and/or early morning awakenings

Insulin resistance: a condition wherein it takes more insulin to drive glucose into the cells, especially when cortisol levels are high

Mild Cognitive Impairment (MCI): a level of cognitive or memory impairment beyond that which usually occurs in individuals normally as they age, but not truly a type of "dementia" or "Alzheimer's disease"

Muscle Atonia: essential muscle flaccidity during sleep, which prevents a person from acting out his/her dreams

Neurogenic Bladder: a malfunctioning urinary bladder due to neurologic dysfunction or insult caused by internal or external trauma, disease, or injury; a neurogenic bladder can cause incomplete emptying of the bladder and make the individual unable to empty the bladder – also known as urinary retention

Nocturia: frequent night-time voiding

Nonpharmacologic interventions: the foundation of care; they include creating a simplistic and safe environment, a predictable routine, counseling for caregivers about the unintentional nature of psychotic symptoms, and offering strategies to manage and cope with troubling behaviors

Orthostatic hypotension: a condition wherein a person's blood pressure drops with positional changes

Prosopagnosia: difficulty recognizing faces

Receptive aphasia: an inability to understand what one is being told

Definitions & Terms

REM sleep: Rapid Eye Movement sleep – the restorative portion of sleep in which a person is dreaming and has rapid eye movement; a person usually has muscle atonia during REM sleep, which prevents the individual from acting out his/her dreams

Sad or Depressed Symptoms: No interest or pleasure in things one used to enjoy, including sex; Feeling sad or numb; Crying easily or for no reason; Feeling slowed down; Feeling worthless or guilty; Change in appetite; Unintended change in weight; Trouble recalling things, concentrating or making decisions; Problems sleeping, or wanting to sleep all of the time; Feeling tired all of the time; Thoughts about death or suicide

Self-neglect: a condition wherein individuals who do not eat right, do not pay attention to personal hygiene, or have issues sleeping – too much or too little, or exhibit behavioral problems

Senility: also referred to as dementia – the loss of mental functions such as thinking, memory, and reasoning, that is severe enough to interfere with a person's ability to carry out the daily tasks of living

Sleep fragmentation: more problems with getting to sleep and staying asleep

Sleep hygiene: go to bed when sleepy, avoid activity in the bed such as reading, watching television, or eating in bed; develop a bedtime ritual; avoid daytime naps; if unable to go to sleep – get out of bed until sleepy

Sundowning behaviors: behavioral problems a person can express, caused by a physiological disease/dementia; these behaviors can include aggression, agitation, apathy, repetitive behaviors, suspicion, and wandering

Urinary incontinence: the involuntary loss of urine

Waddell's sign: when an individual complains of pain, but the pain is not apparent when the person is distracted; pain may indicate a non-organic or a psychological component to chronic low back pain – historically, this has been used to detect "malingering" patients with back pain

Visual hallucinations: seeing abstract shapes or colors or having visions of animals or people that are not really present

APPENDIX A

Opioid Analgesics

Drug	Length of Effectiveness	Comments
Morphine **MS CONTIN** **ORAMORPH**	By intravenous or intramuscular injection: 2-10 mg every 2 to 3 hours Immediate – release by mouth: 3 to 4 hours Controlled – and sustained – release by mouth: 8 to 24 hours	Morphine – MS CONTIN, ORAMORPH – starts to work quickly. The oral form can be very effective for chronic pain. It is more likely to cause itching than other opioids.
Codeine	By mouth: 15-60 mg 3 to 4 hours	Codeine is less potent than morphine – MS CONTIN, ORAMORPH. It is usually taken with aspirin-BAYER – or acetaminophen – TYLENOL.
Fentanyl **SUBLIMAZE** **DURAGESIC**	By mouth: 12-100 mcg Every 3 to 4 hours By patch: 12-100 mcg/24hours applied every 72 hours (3days)	Fentanyl – SUBLIMAZE – lozenges and dissolvable tablets can be used to treat breakthrough pain. Fentanyl – SUBLIMAZE – lozenges can also be used to relieve pain and provide sedation (before painful procedures) in children. A fentanyl – SUBLIMAZE – patch is often used to treat chronic pain.
Hydrocodone **LORTAB**	By mouth: 2.5 to 10 mg Every 4 to 6 hours	Hydrocodone is similar to codeine in effectiveness.
Hydromorphone **DILAUDID**	By intravenous or intramuscular injection: 2-10 mg every 2 to 4 hours By mouth: 2.5 to 10 mg every 4 to 6 hours By rectal suppository: 3-6 mg every 4 hours By mouth: 2.5 to 10 mg every 4 to 6 hours By rectal suppository: 3-6 mg every 4 hours	Hydromorphone – DILAUDID – begins to work quickly. It can be used instead of morphine – MS CONTINORAMORPH – and is useful for chronic pain.

(CONTINUED)

Levorphanol LEVO-DROMORAN	By intravenous or intramuscular injection: 2-3 mg every 4 hours By mouth: 2 mg about every 4 hours	The oral form is strong. It can be used instead of morphine-MS CONTIN, ORAMORPH.
Meperidine	By intravenous or intramuscular injection: 25-100 mg about every 4-6 hours (By mouth: not very effective)	Although meperidine can be effective for short-term use, it is not preferred for long-term use because it has side effects, such as muscle spasms, tremors, seizures, and confusion or psychosis (especially in older people).
Methadone DOLOPHINE	2.5 to 15 mg By mouth: 4 to 6 hours, sometimes much longer	Methadone – DOLOPHINE – is used for treating addiction to heroin and other opioids. It can also be used to treat chronic pain.
Oxycodone OXYCONTIN	5-10mg By mouth: 4 to 6 hours	Oxycodone – OXYCONTIN – can be used instead of morphine – MS CONTIN, ORAMORPH – to treat chronic pain. A long-acting, controlled-release formulation is available, lasting about 8 to 12 hours. The short-acting formulation is usually combined with aspirin – BAYER – or acetaminophen – TYLENOL.
Oxymorphone OPANA	By intravenous or intramuscular injection: 1-1.5 mg every 3 to 4 hours By mouth: 5-10 mg every 12 hours By rectal suppository: 5 mg every 4 hours	Oxymorphone – OPANA – can be used instead of morphine – MS CONTIN, ORAMORPH – to treat chronic pain. Like oxycodone – OXYCONTIN, it is available in a long-acting, controlled-release formulation, lasting about 12 hours.

(CONTINUED)

APPENDIX A - Opioid Analgesics (CONTINUED)

Pentazocine TALWIN	By mouth: up to 4 hours	Pentazocin – TALWIN – can block the pain-relieving action of other opioids. It is about as strong as codeine. The usefulness of pentazocine – TALWIN – is limited because higher doses do not provide more pain relief and because the drug can cause confusion and anxiety, especially in older people. It is not a good choice for older people.
Propoxyphene DARVON	By mouth: 3 to 4 hours	At safe doses, propoxyphene – DARVON – provides little or no more pain relief than aspirin – BAYER. At high doses, it is likely to have side effects. Thus, it is not often used.

(Merck Manual Online-2010)

APPENDIX B

Non-Opioid Analgesics

Acetaminophen is roughly comparable to aspirin in its potential to relieve pain and lower a fever. But unlike NSAIDs, acetaminophen has virtually no useful anti-inflammatory activity, does not affect the blood's ability to clot, and has almost no adverse effects on the stomach. How acetaminophen – TYLENOL – works is not clearly understood.

Acetaminophen is prescribed 325-500mg every 4 to 6 hours as needed – do not exceed 4000mg/24 hours or there is a potential for liver damage/toxicity.

Nonsteroidal Anti-Inflammatory Drugs		
Acetic acid derivatives	*Diclofenac/ Misoprostol* **(Arthrotec)**	50-75 mg twice a day or three times a day
	Diclofenac **(Voltaren,Cataflam)**	50 mg three times a day 150-200 mg daily in 2 to 4 divided doses
	Etodolac (Lodine)	200-500 mg twice a day
	Indomethacin (Indocin)	25-75 mg every 8 to 12 hours
	Ketorolac (Toradol)	20 mg, followed by 10 mg every 4 to 6 hours (Max 40 mg/day) – Elders are at increased incidence of GI bleeding, ulceration, and perforation; also decreased clearance; In cases with renal insufficiency or weight <50 kg – use smaller doses **Note:** The maximum combined duration of treatment (for parenteral and oral) is 5 days – do not increase dose or frequency
	Sulindac (Clinoril)	150-200 mg twice daily or 300-400 mg once daily; not to exceed 400 mg/day
	Tolmetin (Tolectin)	400 mg orally three times a day for 1-2 weeks. Maintenance: 200 to 600 mg orally three times a day. Maximum: 1800 mg/day
Carboxylic acid derivatives	*Diflunisal (Dolobid)*	250-500 mg every 8-12 hours; maximum daily dose: 1.5 g
	Salsalate (Disalcid)	3000 mg/day divided every 8 to 12 hours

(CONTINUED)

APPENDIX B - Nonsteroidal Anti-Inflammatory Drugs (CONTINUED)

Enolic acid (oxicam) derivatives	*Meloxicam (Mobic)*	7.5 mg once daily or twice a day; some patients may receive additional benefit from an increased dose of 15 mg once daily; maximum dose: 15 mg/day
	Piroxicam (Feldene)	10-20 mg/day given once daily or twice a day
Napthylkanone derivatives	*Nabumetone (Relafen)*	500-1000 mg twice a day
Proprionic acid derivatives	*Proprionic acid derivatives*	500-1000 mg twice a day
	Flurbiprofen (Ansaid)	200-300 mg/day in 2 to 4 divided doses. Do not administer more than 100 mg for any single dose; maximum: 300 mg/day
	Ibuprofen (Motrin)	400-800 mg/dose 3-4 times/day (maximum dose: 3200 mg/day)
	Ketoprofen (Orudis)	25-50 mg every 6-8 hours maximum of 300 mg/day
	Naproxen (Naprosyn)	250-500 mg orally twice daily. May increase to 1.5 g/day of naproxen base for limited time period. Controlled release tablet: 375 to 1000 mg orally once daily
	Oxaprozin (Daypro)	600-1200 mg once daily Maximum daily dose: 1800 mg or 26 mg/kg (whichever is lower) in divided doses
COX-2 inhibitors	*Celecoxib (Celebrex)*	100-200 mg twice daily
	Valdecoxib (Bextra)	10 mg once daily

OTHER	
Adjunct Therapies	*antidepressants (such as amitriptyline, bupropion, WELLBUTRIN, desipramine – NORPRAMIN, fluoxetine, PROZAC, and Venlafaxine – EFFEXOR, anticonvulsants (such as gabapentin – NEURONTIN and pregabalin*

APPENDIX C

Non-Narcotic Analgesic Medication

NON-NARCOTIC ANALGESICS	
Fioricet APAP 325mg + butalbital 50mg + caffeine 40mg	1-2 tabs orally every 4 hours (Maximum of 6 tablets/day)
Fiorinal ASA 325mg + butalbital 50mg + caffeine 40mg	1-2 tabs orally every 4 hours. (Maximum of 6 tablets/day)
Soma compound Carisprodol 200mg + ASA 325mg	1-2 tabs orally four times daily
Tramadol Ultram	50-100 mg orally every 4 to 6 hours as needed; max 400 mg/day

OPIATE COMBINATIONS	
Anexsia Hydrocodone/APAP 5/500, 7.5/650, 10/660	1 tab orally every 4 to 6 hours as needed
Darvon Compound Propoxyphene 65mg + ASA 389mg + caffeine 32.4mg	1 tab orally every 4 hours as needed
Lorcet Hydrocodone/APAP 5/500	1-2 tabs orally every 4 to 6 hours as needed (7.5/650 & 10/650): 1 tab orally every 4 to 6 hours as needed
Lortab Hydrocodone/APAP 2.5/500, 5/500	1-2 tabs orally every 4 to 6 hours as needed (7.5/500, 10/500): 1 tab orally every 4 to 6 hours as needed
Percocet Oxycodone 5 mg/APAP 325 mg	1 tab orally every 6 hours as needed
Roxicet Oxycodone/APAP 5/325, 5/500	1 tablet orally every 6 hours as needed

(CONTINUED)

APPENDIX B - *Nonsteroidal Anti-Inflammatory Drugs (CONTINUED)*

Tylenol with Codeine **APAP/codeine** **#2: 300/15,** **#3: 300/30mg,** **#4: 300/60 mg**	1-2 tabs orally every 4 to 6 hours as needed
Tylox **oxycodone 5mg /APAP** **500mg**	1 tab orally every 6 hours as needed
Vicodin **hydrocodone/APAP** **5/500 or Vicodin ES** **7.5/750**	1-2 tabs orally every 4 to 6 hours as needed; Max 8 tablets/day (Vicodin) or max 5 tablets/day (Vicodin ES).
Wygesic **propoxyphene/APAP** **65/650mg**	1 tablet orally every 4 hours as needed

McAuley, D. (2010). Pain Management: The Clinician's Ultimate Reference. Retrieved October 17, 2010. http://www.globalrph.com/pain.htm

About the Author

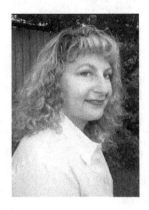

Lisa Byrd, PhD, FNP-BC, GNP-BC, is a seasoned practitioner and gerontologist with a diverse nursing background that includes extensive work in geriatric advanced practice nursing. Dr. Byrd is currently President of Lisa Byrd Healthcare Inc. In this capacity, she oversees physicians and nurse practitioners working at long term care and skilled nursing facilities in several states.

In addition to speaking nationally on a variety of health care topics, Dr Byrd is an Assitant Professor for the University of Mississippi and Adjunct Professor at the University of South Alabama; teaching courses in the graduate nursing programs. She is also a published author, a section editor for Geriatric Nursing Journal, and a successful business owner.

Dr. Byrd shares her expertise with the Alzheimer's Foundation of America as a member of the credentialing team for the "Excellence in Dementia Care Program," offering facility certification in dementia care.